Beyond
Bedlam

Contemporary Women Psychiatric Survivors Speak Out

edited by
Jeanine Grobe

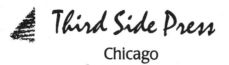

Third Side Press

Chicago

Printed on recycled, acid-free paper in the United States of America. Design and production by Midge Stocker

ATTENTION!
Discontinuing use of psychiatric drugs abruptly can be extremely dangerous—even life threatening—and requires the guidance of a medical professional. The decision to stop any form of therapy or treatment must be made with care. While many of the writers in this book no longer use various psychiatric or psychological services, many still do, and for those who do not, such decisions have often taken years to make and encompass a broad range of specific and individual considerations.This book, while focusing on abuses in the mental health system, is not intended to oppress those individuals who choose those services. Indeed, the purpose of this book is to empower women with psychiatric labels, and that means respecting each of our choices.

Library of Congress Cataloging-in-Publication Data
Beyond bedlam : contemporary women psychiatric survivors speak out /
edited by Jeanine Grobe. — 1st ed.
    p.   cm.
    Includes bibliographical references and index.
    ISBN 1-879427-23-0 (alk. paper). — ISBN 1-879427-22-2 (pbk. :
alk. paper)
    1. Antipsychiatry. 2. Women—Mental health services—Political
aspects. 3. Psychiatric hospital care. 4. Ex-mental patients.
5. Alternatives to psychiatric hospitalization.   I. Grobe, Jeanine,
1957- .
RC437.5.B485   1995
362.2'082—dc20   95-11003
                                                              CIP

Third Side Press
2250 W. Farragut
Chicago, IL 60625-1802

ISBN: 1-879427-22-2 paper   First edition, November 1995
ISBN: 1-879427-23-0 cloth   10 9 8 7 6 5 4 3 2 1

Celia,
Wonderful to
meet you. May
our voices be heard.
Keep up your good work.
Kris

Contents

To Celia –
You are a
strong woman and
I'm proud to know
you. Judi
Chamberlin

Celia, Thanks for being a meddling woman! Pat

iii

ACKNOWLEDGMENTS

My thanks to Myrna Renner, whose faith and friendship have been a warm blanket for my heart; to Cathy Lynn Pagano, who made the sun rise in my life; to my mother and father, for their love.

I would also like to thank my publisher/editor, Midge Stocker, for constant support; creative grace; and most especially, for her integrity and her courage. My thanks to Catherine Odette for introducing me to the psychiatric survivor movement and for her continuing friendship; to Batya Weinbaum, Judi Chamberlin, Barbara Peller, and Sylvia Caras for their help in networking this project. A special thanks to Anne Lawton Lunt for allowing us to use the title *Beyond Bedlam*, the title of her own unpublished book. Finally, my thanks to all of the contributors, each of whom has a permanent place in my heart, and whose suffering and triumph are this book.

PREFACE

Jeanine Grobe

As a woman who has been diagnosed with "mental illness," I honor the blessed courage of all women who have survived this brutal war against ourselves. In addition to surviving our "madness," we've had to survive the "treatment" of our "madness": the solitary cells, the padded rooms, the restraints, the jackets; the forced injections, treatments without consent, commitments against our will; the drugs, electric currents, brain damage; the side effects, broken teeth, spinal injuries, disabilities, deaths, unclaimed bodies buried under numbered plates; the sexual assaults, physical abuse, rapes; the patronizing attitudes, stigmatizing labels, discrimination, invasions of privacy, ostracism, isolation, alienation. The coercion. The scapegoating. The lies that are told against us, the truths that go unheard because we are "paranoid"; the absence of civil rights, human rights, justice. The mangling of mind, body, spirit; the broken parts that never get fixed, the broken lives, the parts forever lost. The pain. The suffering. The world's rejection.

This book is a collection of writings by women who have suffered the stigma and treatment of "mental illness."

Like most people who are products of Western culture, I grew up with the understanding that psychiatry was a branch of medicine like any other. If you had a problem with a tooth, you went to a dentist; if it was your emotions or mental state, you saw a psychiatrist. But after years of "treatment," my understanding changed. I found out that the psychiatric institution was not about healing but about oppression, the oppression of the human spirit. The psychiatric institution taught me to accept being terrorized, tortured, tormented and traumatized because these were "medicine" and I was "sick."

The turning point for me came in 1988 when I began to read the works of radical feminist writers. Through their insights, I realized that there was nothing intrinsically wrong with me; that, in fact, my feelings, experiences, and responses were natural reactions to "wrong" things that were going on around me. As I began to trust my own feelings and instincts, my thought processes cleared, the fragments of my life pieced themselves together and the mystery of my "madness" unravelled. It was soon clear to me that unlike what I had been led to believe, I was not "mentally ill."

What is troubling to those of us who have managed to free ourselves from psychiatric oppression is the awareness that it continues for others. Even more troubling is the knowledge that the society blindly regards psychiatry as safe medicine, a position that is very comfortable since those who reject it are likely to wind up with a psychiatric label themselves. When I began compiling this anthology in 1990, I was unaware that groups of people had already begun speaking out against psychiatry—that an antipsychiatry movement had been in existence since the early 1970s. I only knew that in my seventeen years of involvement with the institution, both as inpatient and as outpatient, oppression had been not the exception but the rule; and that every patient I had been "hospitalized" with was a witness to that truth; and the truth had to be told.

The writings in this book are organized into three main sections:

▲ When the World Can't Face Its Fear, We Get Locked Up
▲ It Doesn't Have To Be Forever
▲ Standing Our Ground: The Political Context of "Madness"

Several lists of resources appear in the appendices at the end of the book, along with biographical notes of the contributors.

▲ ▲ ▲

The writers in this collection represent the countries of Canada, England, Mexico, and the United States. We are women from all classes, races, ages, educational levels, physical capacities, and sexual orientations, presenting a diverse range of perspectives. We all have different faces. Some of us think of ourselves as artists; others, as women with psychiatric disabilities. Some of us think of ourselves as no different than anyone else. What we share is the experience of psychiatric oppression, and in the telling of our experiences, we offer avenues out of it.

Much of the writing here speaks to a suffering shared by both women and men as the diagnosis of "mental illness," and what comes with it affects us all. But, as activist Janet Foner says, women survivors have the "double whammy" of being oppressed both as women, and as women with psychiatric labels. Our voices are rarely heard.

▲ ▲ ▲

Normality is the dominant power group's definition of themselves at a given moment in time. In reality, no one is "normal." But society likes to play the scapegoat game whereby certain groups of people are targeted and claimed to be abnormal, or without worth, or less alive, "not like the rest of us."[*] The purpose of the game is to keep those in power from realizing certain truths about themselves. Where those labeled "mentally ill" are concerned, these truths involve deep, powerful, and often painful insights about the world we live in and have created; thus, it has been universally acceptable to scapegoat the "mentally ill," for it is we who carry the world's pain. And when the pain is too frightening to look at, when it gets too close, when it starts to look like the world's pain, the psychiatric institution provides the service of sealing it (us) off, and keeping it alive.

Bedlam is the popular name for Bethlehem hospital, the first "insane" asylum in England, now notorious for its brutal treatment of mental patients and squalid living conditions. Unfortunately, the inhumane proportions of Bedlam's conditions and treatments are equaled in institutions all over the world today.

But the situation is not hopeless. As the title of this book indicates, the writers here have moved Beyond Bedlam; we the "schizophrenics," we the "manic depressives," have, amidst the clamor of psychiatric jargon, treatment, therapy, and institutions, managed to hear the sound of our own voices. And we're speaking out.

---

[*] See Thomas Szasz, M.D., *The Manufacture of Madness* (New York: Harper & Row, 1970).

But the situation is not hopeless. As the title of this book indicates, the writers here have moved beyond Bedlam; we the "schizophrenics," we the "manic depressives," have, amidst the clamor of psychiatric jargon, treatment and therapy, managed to hear the sound of our own voices. And we're speaking out.

For those readers who have not had direct experience with the psychiatric system, I hope this book will lead you to begin questioning its practices. For the mental health professionals who are reading this book, I hope you will be moved to stand alongside of us as we struggle to end the oppression. For those who are fighters of mental health oppression, may the writings here inspire you to keep going! Finally, for women who are struggling to be free of psychiatric oppression, and for all of you who feel alone in that struggle, this anthology is especially for you. May you find strength in the knowledge that you are not alone, and courage as you read our stories.

PART 1

WHEN THE WORLD CAN'T FACE ITS FEAR, WE GET LOCKED UP

The psychiatric institution is built on the assumption that the experiences of "mad" people don't count—and most of the world has no problem with that. So the suffering involved in being tied to a pole in a vacant ward and allowed to remain there for twenty hours becomes peripheral to what is really important. And your concern about the drug that is causing your breasts to lactate and your menstrual cycles to stop has no power in the "real" world.

Through letters, personal narratives, and diary excerpts, the writing in Part 1 details the events of our lives as mental patients. The writers discuss the circumstances that led to our being institutionalized, "treatment" and other realities in the institution, and living with the stigma. We also discuss our experiences of "madness" without apologizing to the doctors for going above them with our expertise on the subject.

FROM THE INSIDE

Rae E. Unzicker

You wonder how these things begin. Well, this begins in a leafy Kansas town—the kind of place Thornton Wilder created in *Our Town*. Howie the milkman. Mrs. Soames and her gentle gossip. Emily's mother baking cookies. It is the 1950s, a time of television families in which difficult moral dilemmas are presented and resolved in 24 minutes.

Imagine that verdant Midwestern town. The small church college. The town square with the crumbling but still-beautiful county courthouse where ruddy farmers come to retrieve birth certificates, driver's licenses, voter registration cards, tax assessment notices and, finally, documents of death. Lives defined by documents, by the arrogant surety as well as the aching ambiguity of America in the middle of the twentieth century.

In this town there is a street called Cottonwood. All the streets here are named after trees. The town will not outgrow the varieties of trees.

Imagine a talented young girl. A girl who knows she is smart and gifted, who knows, just as surely, that she is different, and that the curse of her differentness will lead to an inevitable clash in a place in which sameness is valued over all other characteristics.

The girl grows, believing—no, *knowing*—that there is something wrong. She is different. She sees things with eyes not yet glazed over with cynicism. She hears music where others do not. She writes lush poems and prose about suffering and about the hurt of being human. She feels, with her eyes, the contradictions of a world that promises protection and provides petty tyranny. Her family is not Jim and Margaret Anderson.

That house on Cottonwood Street where they live is a prison, and she learns to keeps its secrets. Secret injections of drugs. Secret beatings—her parents are proud of these—they "discipline" their child, teach her important lessons. Secret language, somehow spoken sweetly, the language of criticism and judgment, couched in love. We're only trying to help you, they say.

But she knows. She begins to withdraw. Contradictions cause that sometimes.

They love her, they say, and they take her to people who promise help. She is fourteen years old now, and the helpers do not look, do not see, and do not blame. Instead, they give the family a talisman, a magical word that becomes an exoneration. She is sick.

You wonder how these things begin.

▲ ▲ ▲

I remember hearing that word with a kind of relief. Oh, so that's what it is. I'm sick. That explains it. These secret things, these events that are too unspeakable for words have a word, and it belongs to me. I am sick. I need help.

I received help, at least what others called help. My helper sat across a huge brown desk, smoking cigars, accusing, punishing, threatening. No. Helping. I would not—could not—speak. My words were swallowed, or written secretly, only to myself. He gave me drugs, and I swallowed them gratefully. They were merciful in their numbing qualities.

I do not want to be sick. I also cannot live in an environment that makes me sick. I believe I have no choices. Where is the love I was promised? Where is the help I was promised? I want only to die. It is the least I deserve, I believe. And so I try. I wish myself dead, every night. I make what is called an overt attempt. I am caught, and punished for this, too. We punish sick people, they say, smug and self-satisfied.

And still . . .

And still . . .

Go to a hospital, the expert says. They will help you there. You are sick, after all. Sick people belong in hospitals. You wonder how these things begin.

▲ ▲ ▲

I go, my eyes blazing inward with hope. The eyes I allow the
world to see are empty now. Yes, a hospital. Kindness. A doctor
who understands suffering. Rest. I believe. I *must* believe. I am
sick. I need help. The hospital will help.
    And then the final fraud, deception, treachery, betrayal.
Tennyson wrote, "A lie that is half a truth is ever the blackest
of lies."
    I have, finally, discovered the lie, the fraud that is "help" in
a hospital. Help is Thorazine. Ritalin. Mellaril. Help is making
ceramic cups. Help is the day room, day after day after day after
day. Help is volleyball. Help is confinement and imprisonment.
Help is forced labor. Help is learning not to see the violence,
when the very air you breathe is heady with violence. It is the
violence of the milieu; it is what happens when people are
treated as less than human, less than animal. Help is denying the
injustice you see with your own eyes and hear with your own
ears. And always, help is compliance, cooperation, passive
acceptance and, ultimately, gratitude.
    I participate in the lie because I no longer trust my own truth.
I participate willingly.
    I balk only at an attack on my gift, the only thing left that
is truly my own. I am a writer. They called *it*, as well, a lie, a
symptom: grandiosity. No, they say, you are a dishwasher.
No, I say. No. No. NO.
    And I am in seclusion, until I give up this lie to myself and
see that sick people do not write. Sick people wash dishes. We're
only trying to help you, they say.

▲ ▲ ▲

They take my clothes. They leave me naked, without armor.
They lead me, bruising my arms, to the seclusion room, so I can
think about the lie they have given me to live, and change my
mind. The room is remarkable for its starkness. Small, high
ceilings. Dirty white walls smeared with blood and feces and
human suffering. A barred window. A bare light bulb in a cage.
A steel door with no doorknob—click, goes that door—with a
small Plexiglas window through which others—patients, staff,
visitors—cast furtive glances, or openly stare at me, swaddled
in a rough blanket on a cold rubber mattress on a cold concrete

floor. I am cold. So very cold. I smell the fear of the people who
have been here before. Their terror is palpable.

I see things in the silence. I don't cry out my outrage and
disbelief. This is help, after all.

This is what it is to go crazy, I think. Late at night, when the
clouds are still and the moon is high, the memories clamor for
attention. Startled by a moment of clarity in that white room, it
does not seem so bad to go away to other lands inside one's own
mind, to design a refuge from this shame that will now define
my life. No, not mad at all.

You wonder how these things begin.

▲ ▲ ▲

I *did* die there in that room. Oh, I woke, and felt the feel of
dark, not day. What black hours I spent that night, and countless
other nights, in that seclusion room. A part of me is still there,
irretrievable. She is dead. Gone. She was a young woman of
spirit and integrity and hope and vision. She is dead, killed by
the dull lie of help.

I was dragged off, captured in the bright day's savage
madness, overwhelmed by the dark, blind angers of the night;
here, in the sight and sound and smell and feel of the Kansas
prairie, of wheat and sunflowers and the gentle breeze, I was
dragged off to experience a half-death, tortured by what is called
help.

I left that hospital, having washed thousands of dishes, and
having lost my soul.

It did not matter quite so much then, when, several years
later, I woke up in restraints, following a suicide attempt.
Leather cuffs around my ankles and wrists. A leather strap
around my belly. For a moment, just a flicker, I felt the quick,
hot anger. Branded with hate. It left as suddenly as it came. I
had learned. I was sick. I knew how to beg, how to be good. To
lie perfectly still and pretend I was doing it because I wanted to
do it. To understand completely that it was my fault: I had done
something wrong. I deserved to be treated like an animal, to be
humiliated. Of course. I was sick. We're only trying to help, they
say. I lay naked on that bed, a sheet thrown carelessly over me,
and I waited. Recited Shakespeare in my head, oh so quietly, this
dishwasher I had acceded to become.

It did not matter quite so much then, when I was taken to
this prison called a hospital, in handcuffs and leg shackles, and

where I saw—in this "hospital"—another young girl, chained to bedsprings, rattling her pain, using the floor for a toilet.

You wonder how these things begin. These things helpers call "treatment." I will never recover from this. I knew it then. I know it now. You wonder how a system so sophisticated, so technologically advanced, can treat people with such cruelty. Of course, it is not the system at all. It is one doctor, two nurses, an aide, or an orderly. It is *people* who lock people into seclusion rooms, and it is people who affix the leather cuffs or the chains or the gauze strips. It is people who do this and who do not have the courage to confront the unimaginable. It is people who believe they must do what they must do and that what they must do is the expedient thing. It is people who justify torture. "We're only trying to help. We don't know what else to do," they say, with their refrigerated voices.

Does it really matter what else you do? Or is it enough to acknowledge evil, which is indifference to suffering and indifference to the sacredness of the human person? The only way to fight evil is to unmask it, to speak up, to refuse to participate in it, to not be indifferent.

But for us, the hostages of evil, the feeling of endless time is crushing. For us, even when the door is opened, the restraints loosened, we remain captives. We can never forget. We can never really recover.

Each of us remains, in part, a victim of that cruelty, of broken promises, of lies. We are haunted by the memories. The violation permeates our everyday lives. And we are painfully aware of what we have sacrificed:

▲ No longer can you sit for very long in an enclosed car.
▲ No longer can you tolerate light directly in your eyes.
▲ No longer can you be touched without flinching.
▲ No longer is the world a safe place.
▲ No longer do you trust your own clear bright inner voice.
▲ No longer do you believe that help exists.
▲ No longer do you believe that it can never happen to you.
▲ No longer do *you* know what's best for you.
▲ No longer does it ever feel safe to go to a real doctor for a real medical problem.
▲ No longer can you know if you're sad—or if you're depressed. Your feelings—the very essence of you—get questioned, get re-labeled, and the doubt begins. And it is doubt and fear and uncertainty that drive oppression.

What I resent is this: It is not the expediency or even the current fictions of psychiatry. It is the black and hollow lie that is called help.

You wonder how these things begin. And you wonder—oh, how you wonder—how they will ever end.

BECAUSE OF THESE THINGS*

Margaret Robison

Because the old woman
was possibly dying and I said,
"She needs a hand to hold," her breathing
shallow, eyes closed—I was standing
in the hall outside her room
in the insane asylum;
Because of the nurse who was efficient and cruel,
the nurse who sat filling out forms, who rushed
to block the doorway with her body
and I repeated: "I only said
    she needs a hand to hold";
Because the nurse shook a furious finger in my face
and shouted: "You're only a patient
    and don't you ever forget it";
Because of these things, I write
to say that it is true,
I am only a patient
and sixteen years have passed and I
still cannot forget. I cannot forget
the woman who might have been dying
or how roughly two male orderlies
straitjacketed a frightened woman.

I cannot forget her screaming

---

* First appeared in *Sinister Wisdom 36*, Winter 1988/89 issue.

or my own as I lay tied
spread eagle to a bed.
I cannot forget
the macho nurse who stood
scowling as she watched me shower
while I felt helpless and invaded.
(But the water, how grateful I felt then
for the strong rush of water on my skin.)

I cannot forget sitting in a pool
of my own menstrual blood
while visitors came and went and gawked
while I was not permitted
to go down the hall to the bathroom.

There is much I can't forget:
barred windows, pigeons
pecking in the dirt
in the walled-in courtyard, smells
of urine and pine oil,
the stairs to the dining hall,
the greasy stairway railing,
shattered glass on the steps.

I cannot forget
the woman who walked the halls all day
bouncing a red rubber ball—
or occupational therapy
and the woman turned away
because she used profanity; *West Side Story*
on the phonograph, "Somewhere
There's a Place For Us." "Maria."
And the woman who masturbated
in the bathroom with the handle
of the toilet brush. I can never
forget her blank face.

Because of these things, because of the nurse
who said I was only a patient and the woman
who needed a hand to hold,
I have never forgotten.
Nor will I ever forget,

because of the pale hospital walls
with the secrets they hold
of the lives of so many women.
I am amazed those walls stand silent year after year.
I am amazed that blood
doesn't leak through the paint
like a Rorschach
of terrible roses.

WHAT IT IS LIKE TO BE TREATED LIKE A CMI*

Betty Blaska

At the outset, I'd like to say that if we can be called CMIs—chronically mentally ill—then they, the mental health professionals, can be called MHPs. If we must be relegated to a three-letter acronym—and basically stripped of our identity and individuality—then they too can be lumped into one pot. I present a series of vignettes from my history with the mental health system that depict what it feels like to be treated like a CMI.

▲ ▲ ▲

You spend the whole first evening and night crying. You don't want to be here. There must be a mistake. Your only previous experience of this was the movie *Snake Pit*. You're only 18, very young, very naive. You're not yet a CMI. Next day, the "staffing" (as they call it) is very intimidating. All the head brass of the hospital are there. They laugh at you. You tell them you don't want to stay. They patronize you: "Oh, we think we'll keep you a while." You don't know it yet, but you're on your way to becoming a CMI.

---

* First appeared in *Schizophrenia Bulletin*, 17(1), 1991.

▲ ▲ ▲

The first time you experience dystonia from the neuroleptics they've given you, you're extremely frightened. Your tongue is rigid and you're unable to control its movements. You rush to the nurses' station, and they're all huddled inside the little cage's protective walls. They won't leave it for fear of contamination. They are puzzled by your presence and seem greatly inconvenienced by it. You can't speak because of your tongue's movements. Yet they wait impatiently for you to tell them what's wrong. And you wonder what's wrong with them. Can't they see your predicament? But, no. It's not that they don't see. They don't feel. Because you don't count. You're on your way to becoming a CMI.

▲ ▲ ▲

Your first discharge from the psych ward finds you loaded up on major tranquilizers, neuroleptics, and other psychoactive substances. Your follow-up therapist sees you for a while and then announces that he won't continue with you unless you come in with your family for family therapy sessions—all eight of you. But they're scattered all over the state. And they don't want to come in because they hate the shrinks almost as much as you do. They've been belittled, browbeaten, and laughed at by MHPs. So your therapist refuses to see you at all, saying, "If it's important enough for you to see me, you'll get your family to come in." You're not God. You can't get your family to come in. The MHP stops seeing you. And he also refuses to refill the drugs. So you go through withdrawal. And end up back on the same psych ward. And they say to you, accusingly: "Why did you go off your medications?" It's then you realize: you're a CMI.

▲ ▲ ▲

After the second hospital stay, you're supposed to come up with a new MHP to follow you. They send you back to the same clinic where you found the first jerk-therapist. You enter a room, and there are two male MHPs seated in front of you. You ask questions; they look at each other and respond to themselves, not to you. You spend the entire hour having the two shrinks talk *to each other*, not *to you*, but *about you, in front* of you.

At the end of an hour of this frustration, they say they have no openings, that there are no openings in the entire clinic. You wonder why they wasted their time and yours. You wonder who's really crazy—them or you. You start to see more clearly: you're a CMI.

▲ ▲ ▲

During your third hospital stay, one of the MHPs approaches you to inform you that they've asked—demanded—that your parents come in. Today. This afternoon at 1:30. Apparently your parents have replied that they couldn't. It was the first good planting day and your dad was in the fields. The MHP informs you that the hospital threatened to send you to a big state mental institution, if your parents didn't come in. You express indignation at their ultimatum and defend your parents. They have six kids. You're one of them, but your father has to put food on the table for eight people. The MHPs seem alarmed by your defense of your parents. Well, their threat worked: your parents are there that afternoon. Now the MHPs haughtily announce that they've changed their minds. They're sending you to a state mental hospital anyway. Your defense of your father was an "admission" that you feel less important than the rest of your family. Your lack of self-esteem is deplorable.

The lesson? A CMI, even a CMI's family, is powerless next to one or more MHPs. Your parents discharge you AMA (against medical advice) from the clutches of this hospital's self-righteous MHPs. The MHPs' pronouncement of your "low self-esteem" is their first lesson in doubting your own basic instincts.

▲ ▲ ▲

The next MHP you get hooked up with is a loony. The less said about him the better. Except that he gets fired some months after you quit seeing him—for alcoholism—and you're not surprised at that.

▲ ▲ ▲

You're sitting in a huge lecture hall in a medical school where first-year med students are receiving their first psychiatry lecture. You're taking the course as part of graduate studies, and you're in a depressive phase. A woman who is an inpatient of the psych ward is being interviewed. The uneducated and uninformed medical students find her delusions "funny" and do not hide their laughter but display it openly. You try to hide your crying. But it's not only tears for you or for the woman. The tears are for these future MHPs who will never acquire the education or insight or sensitivity they need to help heal the CMIs in their world.

▲ ▲ ▲

Then you end up in Psychopathic Hospital—don't you love the title? There they tell you you were misdiagnosed. You find out you're not schizophrenic, you're manic-depressive. You tell the new MHPs that the former MHPs sued you for a $3,366.66 bill. They sent the sheriff after you with a subpoena. That you want to sue *them*. Would the new MHPs testify that you'd been misdiagnosed and mistreated—treated with the wrong medications—your symptoms made worse, not better? Oh, no! They wouldn't consider testifying against fellow shrinks. Who knows! Someday they might be sued. They have a collegial loyalty to each other. Their reputations are on the line. Their salaries are at stake.

And who are you? One little patient, one little CMI!

▲ ▲ ▲

As an inpatient in what's called a "mental institution" you go to something they call OT—occupational therapy. Everything here is called *therapy*—even when it isn't.

And today it's "assertiveness" class! Whoopie! Someone back in the 1960s decided that the hallmark of a mentally healthy person was being assertively able to choose and refuse, speak, act, and listen. This is a mockery inside a place called a "mental institution," because here no mental patient is free to choose, refuse, speak, or act. You can't even listen to each other without someone spying, reporting, recording, and charting. And then calling you paranoid if you notice. Or object.

And when you refuse an activity or "therapy"—which they tell you is your right—and which they've taught you to do in their "assertiveness" class, then they badger you by sending nurse after nurse, attendant after attendant, into your room to remind you that "It's 1:00. Time for OT!" Your refusals mean nothing. They badger you until you either give in and go, or they've frustrated you to tears. Or enraged you to anger. And then they can justify calling you by the malignant label they've designated you by—resisting treatment or "noncompliant," passive dependent, passive aggressive, paranoid, or borderline personality disorder. They're all different labels. But they all mean the same thing: you're not really you. You're just a CMI. And that justifies the MHP's dehumanization of you.

▲ ▲ ▲

You've been in and out of the hospital, on and off a cadre of psychoactive drugs. In doses you complain are too high. In combinations you complain are too much. A year and a half of being some high-priced pseudoscientist's guinea pig. (I've always contended that *he* should pay *you*—not the other way around—for the privilege of trying out the latest psychopharmaceutical fad on you.)

And of course you've lost your job. Who could work amid all this drug experimentation? And the myriad of drug side effects—nausea, diarrhea, dizziness. Vision so bad you can't cross the street because you can't judge the cars' distance from you. Drug-induced psychosis so bad you can't leave your bed or look out the window for the terror you feel. Blood pressure so low you can't stand for very long, and your voice so weak you can't be heard across a telephone wire.

So you're without a job. And they send you to a place called DVR—Division of Vocational Rehabilitation. They "help" you get a clerical job. Never mind that you don't want to do that kind of work. Never mind that you have a degree—or two. Or that you have dreams. They "help" you get a clerical job because, yes, you've guessed it, you're a CMI. A woman CMI. But the men CMIs are just as lucky. They get to become janitors!

▲ ▲ ▲

You're depressed. You're feeling suicidal. None of the medications is working. The blackness ushers in suicidal ideation almost without your needing to give any conscious direction to your thoughts. Your thoughts—they're all negative. Trying to steer them into something positive—because they've said cognitive therapy works!—only ends in bringing up something negative along with it. You catch the negative thought and start over with something new, until it, too, leapfrogs you into another negative one. It's as if a whole Pandora's box has opened in the attic of your mind, only that box is labeled "black." And the box labeled "white" is locked tight, the key thrown away. And you tire of this endless exercise of redirecting the thoughts. Your mind, nerves, and body are fatigued enough as it is.

You call a place named Crisis Intervention Services. The person who answers is brusque and unkind. She adds more stressors to your already overtaxed nervous system. You don't want to go on with this life. You're told your situation is not serious enough. And besides, she doesn't have time for you. You feel insignificant. You are. You're a CMI. And you're only one CMI in a county with 1,500 CMIs.

▲ ▲ ▲

You have a cyclical disorder. After the second year at the same job and the second episode, your MHP tells you it would be better if you worked part-time. You know you can work more than full-time when you're well, which is three-fourths of the year, and you can't work at all when you're ill, which is one-fourth of the year. But he's the MHP, so you go along.

Now you're working for the state; they encourage accommodating for the handicapped, and you guess you're one of these. And you're working at a typist classification, for which job-sharing and finding another typist to work the other half-time should be a cinch. But your boss happens to be a big-shot neonatologist. He insists they need *one full-time* typist. He won't budge. And the medical school won't budge. And their affirmative action officer can't make him budge. So you're forced out of the job. It's then you're reminded: you're only a CMI.

▲ ▲ ▲

You have severe abdominal pains again in the middle of the night. The last time the Emergency Room (ER) doctor said to come over right away when you get the pains to better diagnose them. So you go. A different ER doctor is there. He asks you the preliminary questions. Then he comes to "Are you taking any medications?" After you name the psychotropic drugs you're on, his face changes to one of skepticism. Suddenly he doesn't believe the pains are real. He finds nothing in his examination. And he says he doesn't have any notes from any other ER doctor (though your last visit was only a week ago). He doesn't believe you. You're malingering, or hypochondriacal, or psychotic, or worse. You know the truth. But the truth can't be believed: you're only a CMI.

▲ ▲ ▲

You file a sexual assault grievance against an MHP. The investigation is as painful as the episode, and you are depressed for days. But the examining board finds in his favor. You get the transcripts of the testimony. It's said that you have a personality disorder (news to you). It's said you put people in no-win situations. But, *he* wins the suit and you've been losing all your life. It's his word against yours, and you have a psychiatric label. He's the respected professional; you're only a CMI.

▲ ▲ ▲

What have you learned as a CMI? Abuse—physical, emotional, spiritual, sexual, and financial; humiliation; belittlement; vulnerability; lack of credibility. Reduced to a three-letter acronym; stripped of dignity; denied your own inner conviction, feeling, and instincts; frustrated; stigmatized; expected to conform; always wrong; put in double binds; given a lack of choice; lack of control; and lack of love; left with nothing; and finding it's better not to feel, not to try, and even not to live. Until today.

Today you speak out. Today you reclaim yourself. Today you begin to heal, to heal others. Today you educate others and reeducate still others. Today life begins anew for you and for others whose consciousness you are trying to raise. Today the patient, ex-patient, mental health consumer movement is reclaiming the dignity and power of the CMIs of this world.

INSOMNIAC

Elaine Erickson

A man is lodged in my brain.
He talks and talks—an ant
moving in circles. He calls
my finest dream a burned-out
racehorse. He breathes
his black gas in my brain
and I pour sadness at his feet.
He pulls a shower curtain over his eyes
when I cry. If I tell him
I love him, he tells me I am one of many.
If I tell him I hate him, he's a curse.
I want to believe
in miracles. I like to think
I could lie with him in peace,
cotton candy stuffed in our mouths,
our words inching away
like quivering worms.
But he's always there talking,
his words busy traffic climbing
cell upon cell, tumbling
blocks of thoughts, scattering, plundering
the landscape of my mind.

I will kill him.
I will smother him, his words squeaking out
like rubber pennies. Then I will turn over
in my bed and reach for the lamp,
switching it into darkness.

THE SHOCKING TRUTH

(For Susan)

Dorothy Washburn Dundas

I can still feel the cold, sticky linoleum beneath my bare feet as I shuffled my way to the bathroom on those freezing early mornings during the winter of 1960. The sensations and memories are as much a part of me now as they were then, perhaps even more vivid now, as I realize the shocking brutality of my treatment as an adolescent girl locked into a mental institution because of my overwhelming feelings of depression.

We were lined up side by side in our beds on those mornings, four girls, huddled beneath our cold, white sheets, petrified and silent. I can see the nurse in her starched white uniform. I can smell the alcohol she rubbed on my bottom, and I can feel the sting of the sharp needle as she injected the insulin into me: insulin coma therapy, five days a week for six weeks.

After we were groggy from the insulin, but often not yet in a coma, the second treatment would begin. I can still see him walking through the door to our bare hospital-green room, his face, gray-white in color, and his black suit and black shoes. He carried all his equipment in a small black suitcase in one hand, this man of death and destruction. He set up his machine behind our heads, one by one. Curled up beneath our sheets, heads covered, as though seeking womb-like protection, we were, as they peeled the sheets off us, one by one, forcing us onto our backs, bare and open and vulnerable. I was second in the line-up.

Before being turned, I would often peek out from a small, secret opening in my sheet to see what they were doing to Susan, the first to receive the treatment. I would make myself watch as if it might prepare me in some way. And when she would shake

33

violently all over, my eyes would close. I could no longer watch. I would shiver beneath my sheet in fear. And then they would come to me. I can still feel the sticky, cold jelly they put on my temples. My arms and legs were held down. Each time, I expected I would die. I did not feel the current running through me. I did wake up with a violent headache and nausea every time. My mind was blurred. And I permanently lost eight months of my memory for events preceding the shock treatments. I also lost my self-esteem. I had been beaten down.

But I was lucky. I was very, very lucky. On one of those cold winter mornings exactly thirty years ago, they injected my friend, Susan, in the bed next to me, with more insulin than her frail young body could tolerate. A few hours later, as the four of us were having our mandatory afternoon nap, still huddled beneath our sheets, my friend Susan went to sleep and never woke up. She had just turned seventeen. When she died, she became a part of me.

On the winter afternoons after Susan died, I can remember my "mental health care" continued by my being taken into that same shock room, where we also slept at night, by a mental health worker. He would lock the door, push me up against the wall, and sexually abuse me. My head foggy from the insulin, dazed from the drugs, I was petrified. I did not scream. I did not dare. I survived. And I did not tell anyone for a long, long time.

▲ ▲ ▲

After six months, I was transferred to another institution. What I recall most vividly from that institution is the seclusion. The room was dark and hot and sticky. It was bare except for the roughly covered, striped mattress. There was no sheet. I could feel every thread in the fabric against my skin as if I were being cut into pieces with my every move. And inside, the pain was rushing through my head and every vein. I could feel the Thorazine sting as they injected the needle into my skin, and I would then become a stranger to myself, dead and dying from the inside out. It went on for weeks and weeks and weeks. I was crying for Susan, for my shattered self, for my lost freedom. I was trying to survive. The seclusion did not help. And the drugs nearly killed me.

One woman I shall always remember for her fearless rage. In her fifties, she wore her graying black hair pulled tightly back in a bun, and she always wore the same long, dark, straight dress and black shoes with thick high heels. Her fury was something to behold. The only times I saw this amazing woman were when she would emerge from her room, three times a day, tray in hand, and smash the entire tray with all the food spraying upside-down across the floor outside her door, screaming that she did not want to be locked up and she would not eat the food until they let her go free. Her shrieks were piercing, sometimes even frightening; but I always held her in very high esteem because of her bravery and her ability to yell out the truth before all of us who were much younger and much more afraid.

During the three years I spent in institutions, I saw and experienced a lot of abuse. Some of it was violent, some of it was more subtle, but it was almost always present in one form or another, like a polluted river running through our lives. We did the best we could to survive. Many of us did not. We were all thought of as crazy when, in fact, we were trying desperately to adapt to a societally sanctioned form of control under the guise of "mental health care." Most of us were in a war, not only a war within ourselves, but also a war against the system that had put us there. And it was not a war we could ever win. We tried and tried and tried.

▲ ▲ ▲

I learned a lot from my experiences. One thing I learned was never to remain silent in the face of abuse. I also learned that the least restrictive, personal, and compassionate care most often leads to healing. After I was released from the last institution, I was fortunate finally to find that rare and healing kind of care, which enabled me, in spite of my experiences, to rebuild my life.

Recently, I attended a hearing before Judge Rya Zobel in U.S. District Court where I heard horrifying stories of neglect, overuse of restraint, medication, and seclusion.* A nurse told of elderly women tied to their beds for hours on end because there

---

* *McNamara vs. Dukakis.* Relatives and friends of Massachusetts' nearly 5,000 mental patients filed suit seeking restoration of funding that was reduced through budget cuts ordered by Governor Michael Dukakis. According to the suit, the cuts "expose many patients to risk of serious physical harm, unnecessary restraint, and hospitalization."

were not enough nurses to care for them properly. I remember women such as those she described. Sitting in that courtroom, as I heard the witnesses testifying on behalf of the patients, the pictures in my mind from thirty years ago became clear, Technicolor crisp, with intricate detail: The old women were lined up and tied to their chairs from 6 a.m. until 8 p.m. They mumbled in the hall next to each other. Sometimes they wailed and pleaded to be let out. They wore diapers, and their urine often spilled out onto the floor. I tried to soothe them; they were inconsolable. They were the women who had been abused in their youth; many had been shocked, overmedicated, secluded for years. They were the women who never made it out. They were a constant reminder of what could happen to all of us who were so much younger. They were the old women of thirty years ago, now dead. The old women of today are still tied to their beds. In many, many cases, their "illnesses" have been caused by the atrocities within the system over the years. I saw it happen.

It is important to know that the worst atrocities happened to me in the prettiest places. One looked like a farmhouse from the front, with lots of flowers and trees. Way back in the woods, there was a small concrete unit where the shock patients were housed. That was where I spent most of my time. The other pretty hospital looked like a college campus. At least no one pretended that the state hospitals looked like a college campus. At least no one pretended that the state hospitals were pleasant. They looked horrible, and they were horrible. The "nice" places were an illusion where more drugging and sexual and physical abuse happened to me than anywhere else.

SAINT CECELIA

Elaine Erickson

The beauty operator turns Cecelia's hair
to gold—a maze
of mirrors and smiles.

Cecelia walks down the street proudly,
the sun trapped in her hair
like a brilliant white fish.
Now she shivers to a thread, a squawking
of horns—then corridors of blue
through morning clouds, a sea gull's
merciful cry. Suddenly

she is lost in an ink well
of blackness. Hall lights glimmer
like goldfish. She opens a door.
A frightening choir of sneering faces,
a smear of neon lights.
She hesitates, like a high diver ready to plunge.
"Why are you here?" asks a woman behind a desk,
her eyes pools of steel.
"A blood test," mumbles Cecelia.
"What is your diagnosis?"
The faces stare.

Cecelia is in a pasture, a clumsy cow
kissing her fingers. She lowers her voice.
"Schizophrenia."
"Go sit with the others," the woman snarls,
swirling around in her swivel chair.

MIND CONTROL

Anne C. Woodlen

I'm fairly militant on the subject of mental illness. I make no bones about the fact that I have a mental illness and am, like a good grave site, in perpetual care. I refuse to let society make me feel any more ashamed of having borderline personality disorder than of having pneumonia. I'm glad I don't have something *really* embarrassing like hemorrhoids, but, be that as it may, some things just defy a humorous recounting. My last hospitalization, for example.

The memory of this hospitalization causes me great pain and a goodly amount of fear. What do you, as a friend, want to know? What do you, as a taxpayer, have the right to know? What do you, as a citizen, have the responsibility to know? I was admitted to a state psychiatric center in New York with a pre-existing broken leg—in February 1992.

The Doctors

Dr. A saw me first, and told me she was holding me over for Dr. B's return from vacation. Dr. B saw me, but said that Dr. A was my doctor. Dr. A went on vacation after saying that Dr. C was my doctor. Dr. B saw me again but said that Dr. C was my doctor; Dr. C said Dr. A was.

They behaved with all the grace and maturity of the three stooges: Curly pokes Larry in the eyes, Moe smacks Curly with a frying pan, and Larry loses his pants. This A-to-B-to-C routine would have been funny were it not that my life and freedom were at stake.

The Chili-Bowl Referral

There are two meals that the hospital does superbly. One is chili and the other is spaghetti. I had just sat down to a chili lunch when Dr. C and the social worker showed up. It was immediately evident that they expected me to abandon my meal and go elsewhere to meet with them, but I was not about to blow one of the two decent meals I would get out of the sixty or so that I would be served; if the roles had been reversed and Dr. C were doing the eating and I wanted to do the talking, would she interrupt her meal for me? In a pig's eye.

So I sat my ground, and they decided to sit down at my table, which blew the program for the rest of the diners. There were not enough seats for the patients, but that didn't seem to bother Dr. C and the social worker.

They sat and told me that I was to ship out on Friday for the first of a two-day trial at a continuing treatment unit. I wanted to ask why and what for, but in my chastened state all I could do was mumble agreement. They gave me no reason or rationale for the referral. Just do it, they said; okay, I said.

Four-Point

The patient is moved to the third floor, and four-point. Dr. D told me he hated putting people in four-point. Certainly people hated being put in four-point; nevertheless, the system designed and built a special room for four-point. It is not a kind of needlepoint or a geographical heading or a place in the band. It means being tied hand and foot to a bed. Call it four-point. Pretend reality is not what it is. This is a psychiatric ward.

Tied-hand-and-foot is not reserved for six-foot hulks who are violent and frighten everybody; it is matter-of-factly used on a 98-pound woman with anorexia.

It is just this year that they have installed the tied-hand-and-foot room. It is not a remnant of prehistoric psychiatry; it is state of the art. Why is the system regressing? What's next? Being chained to the wall in a dungeon? Call it stellar cellar therapy.

Censorship

I was getting no scheduled individual therapy, no group therapy, and no passes. In despair, I called old weird Stan over in the Education Department and asked him to go to the library and seek out for me some literature on the subject of borderline personality disorder; if I had to commit self-therapy, I would.

Stan was quite willing, but noted that he was currently in hot water with a bunch of doctors and—if his boss recommended it—would I mind if he went through the motions of clearing it with my doctor? Of course not; I understood. So Stan went to Jonathon, and Jonathon said he should ask Dr. C, so Stan did. Dr. C said he could not bring me any material; he could, however, bring material to her and she would screen it.

My father was a college professor. In the home I grew up in there was a room called "the library." It contained hundreds of books. I have always assumed that the free movement of ideas on paper was an elemental right. And that one thing one could be proud of was one's openness to new or different ideas. To be denied free access to books fills me with terror. And please remember the context in which this happened: I was in a locked psychiatric ward, being denied passes. I was, finally, being denied freedom of thought.

Dr. C, when I confronted her, used the word "like." I would be permitted to have material if she liked it.

What do you do with a mental health system in which one person has the power to deny ideas to another person? I indict Dr. C for attempted mind control.

Stanley, however, gets cheers and orchids and assorted kudos for being a guerrilla fighter in the war for freedom of the mind: he photocopied the title pages of the books that he gave to Dr. C, as well as photocopying a borderline personality disorder article in a professional journal. When Stan came to see me on the locked ward, he took me to the end of the nearly-deserted sunroom, hugged me, and slid the photocopied material into my hand, muttering laughingly, "If you're captured, eat this!"

THE SILENT ONE*

Myrna Renner

My Parents

After all these years I still wonder why you put me here (what harm could a five-year-old do).

You brought me here to this man-made hell (never to come back for me).

I don't remember what you look like anymore (if I ever see you again, I will kill you).

Not for bringing me here, but for never telling me why.

What harm could a five-year-old do?

I wonder if you think of me or have you forgotten the child you locked away—I'm grown now, and still here. I still wonder why you did what you did, but I'll never know—as you're outside and I'm in here.

The Dreamer

You stare out the bars day after day (I wonder what you see out there).

You gaze into a world that isn't even there (the bars will keep you here even if you want to run).

Your mind must cover miles, as you stand there for hours (I wonder where you travel, when you look past these bars).

Do you travel to places we'll never go?

---

* These selections are from *The Silent One*, a collection of prose poems published by the author.

Do you see things we'll never see?

Do you ever go beyond the bars to a place where there is peace? (Someday the bars will fall and you can run free.)

You stare out the bars day after day. Wherever you go, stay awhile as you look peaceful, and you escape from here a while if only in your mind.

State Inspection

It must be inspection time again as the floors are getting mopped and waxed and staff is going crazy trying to cover their ass.

It must be inspection time again as we've all been given clean sheets and a blanket (it will disappear when this is over).

It's kind of fun to watch staff running around in circles and trying to get their paperwork done and in order (probably hasn't been done in months).

It must be inspection time again as we are all getting deliced and haircuts (any other time they wouldn't care if the bugs were jumping off us, nor our hair in order). We all smell like disinfectant.

It must be inspection time again—only nice thing about it—we don't have to eat oatmeal today and we'll get real food.

Well, it's time for the show to begin: the inspectors are here (let the games begin, first the tour, then the kitchen, and then comes us).

We know better than to talk or move from our chairs. If we do, there will be hell to pay later (I wonder what would happen if they knew the truth about this place).

Inspection team is leaving, we can move around now and talk but we better pray they passed or we'll be sorry (someday, I will tell the truth about this hell hole and the ones that run it). SOMEDAY!

A Bad Day

It's going to be a bad day. The nurses are too busy to unshackle us from our beds (I hope I don't have to go to the bathroom).

It's going to be a bad day. The bitch is on duty again (we'll never get up now, until it suits her).

Everyone is starting to yell and scream. They've been shackled down long enough (she says that if we'll be quiet and settle down, we can get up in an hour).

The ward is starting to smell and the odor is making me sick (somebody had to go to the bathroom; they'll have a lot of beds to change before this day is over).

It's going to be a bad day. As long as we're shackled down, they have control and know where we are (no need for bed count today: we're all in them).

Well, she just let us up, but she got paid back for keeping us down; Mike just threw shit all over her (not such a bad day after all).

Weekend Pass

The doctors have given everyone weekend passes. You would think after all these years I would get used to it (I keep hoping, someday, someone will come and get me, so I can go too).

Everyone's excited about going home for a few days (freedom) and they're busy packing (I'll watch them leave through the window and keep smiling).

Family after family comes, and one by one, they leave (they don't even say good-bye anymore as they know I'll be here when they return; someday I'll get to go, someday).

You'd think I would just accept it—they all go and I stay—but I keep dreaming that someone will come and say I can go with them (I don't care who, just someone).

They've all gone now. I have the whole place to myself, except for the crazy one in the chair (I think I'll go see if he wants to play pattycake, he's a simple-minded thing).

They've all gone now—it's just me and the crazy one and staff. They've given me freedom in the day room to do what I want (I'll ask the crazy one if he wants to fingerpaint the walls).

They all have gone now. I wonder what they do out there for three days (no matter, I'll hear about it all Sunday; that's the hard part, as they all have something to tell and I have nothing to say).

Someday that doctor is going to give me a pass and when he does, you can bet your ass I'm going and I'm taking the crazy one with me, one way or the other, as he has been here with me every weekend for years and I won't leave him here by himself (if he can't go, we'll stay behind, but we'll be together).

Lobotomy

They have taken you out in the night because you were screaming (I will watch your bed until you get back).

They took you out in the night; it's been days now and no sign of you (I'm frightened for you; none of us can find you and we've looked everywhere).

They took you out in the night. It's been too long now and you've not returned to your bed (I've been watching staff like a hawk and nothing).

They have just brought you back and put you in your bed and left (my God what have they done to you—your eyes are blank, your head is wrapped, and your body limp).

They have made you a vegetable like the others, never again to know who I am and that I will miss you.

Caretakers and Shock Treatment

You took my mind, destroyed whoever I was, and left me lost in a world I don't know and with a person I have no knowledge of—and you expect me to live with a stranger within myself and survive.

You stripped me of my name and replaced it with a number; you erased what memories I had of life and told me things I have to believe or I have nothing.

I trusted you like a child, believing you would care for me in my insanity and silence, awakening to find out you destroyed me and made me an outcast even to myself.

Free Day

Today was my first day of real freedom (I was gone for a whole day with real people).

I saw a man playing a horn on the street (playing for his sweetheart, because it's Valentine's Day).

I ate at a place with my friend where there were no orders of where to sit and what to eat (I ate what I wanted).

My friend got me some glasses so I could see better (maybe the world will look different to me now, and I can see the flowers bloom in spring).

I have a new friend in my life. She's a normal person, but it doesn't matter to her that I'm a little different (she lets me be me).

It's been a different day. I have run away from insanity for a little while only to realize there is a world outside of here and someday I am going to go there.

sometimes i fall forever downward toward an end

Beth Greenspan

sometimes i fall forever downward toward an end

sometimes the haze is black and thick, filled with
    week-old
coffee grounds, and i o.d. on the blackness, the void and
    caffeine-filled
overwhelming sense of mixed direction signs leading fast
    and aimlessly
toward the edge, the edge past my office window that i
    can't even see
out of; the densified air turned to cloudy crystals that drift
    down
if you knock on it and this is my brain as i stare into it,
    forcing
my eyes to stay open, somehow connected, lost, forever
    the paranoid wanderer
looking for home, a place to rest thoughts, fleshy
    coexistence between
what i am and what i can't get out of; and if you ask me
    to talk, i do,
but i cannot really tell you the story because it
    encompasses the earth,
life and death mistakenly identified as the same creature
    and, no, you
cannot realize because i cannot realize but i thank you for
    whatever you
have given and i hope i did not bring you closer to the
    truth.

sometimes to move is scary, to stay still is scary, watching
    the strange faces
watch me and i'm very scared of this world, very scared
    of me, because i embody
something i cannot explain, an end-filled idea so
    confusing like watching
a storm come, then go, knowing it will come again and
    never knowing when,
never knowing how it moves, breathes, never knowing
    the complete details
of its existence, and with the devastating fear, the
    tear-filled eyes alone,
i can't do all of what you ask me to do, with one minute
    floating on after
another, after another, i cannot do what you ask me to do
    because there is
a certain lostness in this universe, lives within lives within
    deaths within
lives and everyone says i can't expect miracles, nor
    answers, but then how to go about what everyone else
    calls life?

sometimes, often, i just end up distantly staring at the
    comings and goings
of others and wish, how i wish for something else; peace
    of mind? guidance?
an end? to what? love? sometimes just walking to get
    somewhere, anywhere, home,
seems an impossible task and was it meant to be and i've
    lost you so why am
i asking if all i can hear is the screaming of misfits in my
    head? sometimes
someone asks what this is and i say it is just that, but really
    it is a painful
echo all around of all the lost and hiding ones like me who
    are screaming
for . . .

sometimes there is no reason to wait but i do anyway,
    half-expecting mother

to come and put me back in her womb, half-expecting the
    world to explode
at any moment, half-expecting me to implode toward a
    very tiny center
of golden flames like the phoenix going backward into
    the earth to the core;
half-expecting you to fully comprehend the situation but
    in person i can do
no more but say hello, goodbye, goodbye to the end of
    this day and sometimes
there follows another and one after that and when it is all
    over, the sunset
after the rain, we laugh at the chaos, but now i cry because
    it isn't over,
i am just a bad dream, i am the nightmare that wraps itself
    around my throat
and pulls me down, further and further lost from the day
    and all the time
trying to explain is not even worth these words and all
    the time there is
the panicked exhaustion of feeling this is it, last train
    going out past
midnight, crashing into air at the end of the line and then
    i crash into
morning, afraid of darkness and light, heavy terror of
    worldly remembering and . . .
i swallow the pill.

BEYOND BEDLAM[*]

Anne Lawton Lunt

The back ward was something else. No horror movie ever prepared her for this reality.

Her body's energy was sapped from sleepless nights, the flesh stripped from days of fasting, her mind impotent to clear a way amidst the walls with no end. Vulnerable now to the fright her eyes drew into her, the sounds her ears felt, the smells past stench, and the worst possibility of all, the death of the spirit, her soul screamed, "Could God possibly be here?"

My God, My God. Rows of beds, white on white, antiseptic fumes permeated the atmosphere. Urine and feces, barely masked, hovered around the edges. Wrinkled ghosts of days long past walked in shuffles between the aisles of beds, mouthing their familiar litanies, their identities of repetition. Clothed in sacks of drabness, lost in a sea bound by the shores of steel-grated windows, they populated the porch with no chairs.

The benches cold, like the purple legs of the "dumb one" standing mute, head hung down, strings of hair hung like a dirty floor mop, the face idiotic. Ramblings of children chattering alone, or to another, deaf to there, that place with no heart beating, beating. Jibber, jabbering, jibber jabbering. Sounds, swaying bodies, purposeless going nowhere business. Bare living. Lightly animated vegetables. Not quite. Just looks that way.

---

[*] This is an excerpt from an unpublished manuscript entitled *Beyond Bedlam.*

A bathroom right there, with no door. Open stalls for four or five, some bowls, and a couple of mirrors. A place to take a walk, look in the glass, see a face, and wonder who is that in there. That gaunt, hollow-eyed cadaver, breathing in a nameless nightmare.

No one to talk to. The toll of the past days taking its price. They feed these people something. Like a trough of leftovers. She was so sick with this, and all that came before it, she refused her dinner. They told her, warned her, she must eat. They would help her and stuff it down her nose with tubes, and do it that way every time if she refused. She was so frightened, she agreed to eat when she knew she couldn't. She threw up all over the clean johnny she had on to wear. She was so sorry for this, she apologized to the attendants, all in tears, and said she'd wash it out. Compliant now, from the first loss of hope, her first struggle to please, to conform to the reality of this place, squelched, she became aware of where she might be. It wasn't good to see.

This back ward was the testing ground. They watched her for several days for any violent acting out, or intense behavior.

The nights were short, or long, depending on her inner turmoil. Since it was the catacomb of the living dead, the lights stayed on nearly all the time. They went off early, and came on at three or four in the morning. All these bodies in the beds had lights in their faces, and darkness outside.

Food was served before dawn. It didn't matter. How could a turnip or a carrot care what time it got watered, or when the artificial sun came on? What difference did it make to them?

Vegetables can say words. She was so lonely, she talked to these people, or these shells of people.

They called it a women's ward. Maybe they had been women once, or, maybe no one ever knew what one was. It certainly seemed this place was full of whatever they were.

Maybe they were no good, and someone put them here. What crimes did they commit? Wandering around between the aisles, a punishment for life. No sun anywhere. Their reality was the teddy bear they once had. Fragments of lives mouthed to thin air in repetition of the familiar. Like so many frail anchors to a life choked off, these words from shapeless dresses and matted hair.

She found the words of each, intruded herself into everyone possible, and had many conversations with the fragments of many broken lives, and one would daresay, hearts.

Many hours were passed this way. Other times she spent on the porch, staring at the remnants of human life congregated out there in some haphazard way. Some of them were sitting stuck in rigid positions, some stiff, some moving about. Red and purple legs. Puddles of urine to step over, rocking, swaying, people excuses. Murdered hearts and souls robbed of dignity, warehoused animal cadavers, cared for by the robot machines of a specimen-oriented world.

She talked at them, shouted at them. She looked at them hard. She was very angry at them for being that way, for letting that happen. She was very angry for the nameless, faceless demons who pushed them into their cauldron of inhuman dimensions.

She was mean sometimes. She had nothing to do but watch and stare and strive to incite some responses from these other fellows in this macabre zoo. She was nice a lot. Why not? They were in it together. Victims of their fellows.

They were women. Could that be possible? But then, she had no idea what a woman was!

ATTACK

Beth Greenspan

If I had a door
You would not be able to see me
Curled in a ball hands covering eyes
And you wouldn't be able to whisper
"She's losing it"
To the others who infrequently stare
As they pass by this unsolitary place
While my brain storms and burns holes
Through passing time
And although the kinder of you
Wishes there were something you could do
Fear of the unknown and chancy misunderstandings
Leave your reactions and abandonments up to instinct.
This is a temporary situation
But it will hit again.
This is a temporary situation
And the way you are can cause it.
This is a temporary situation.
Repeat.

STRUGGLING TO BE BORN[*]

Judi Chamberlin

Was it purposeful or just force of circumstance? The world wasn't really conspiring to drive me crazy; it was just accident that loving parents, concerned educators, and healing doctors had precisely that effect. Just as ineffectually as the single soldier who claims that it's everyone else who is out of step, I struggled against everyone else's conception of what I was and what I should become.

The first enemy was education. Longing to escape the rote and regimentation, I retreated into daydream and fantasy. What would have been accepted in a dull child was heresy in a bright one (and didn't they have my I.Q. score to blind them to seeing the very real and confused child?). What I needed was the opportunity to wander, to adventure, to question, and to learn—but there were no free schools then, and the city was far too dangerous a place for a child to be allowed to roam freely. The choices were narrow: conformity, which brought a pain that must be hidden, or rebellion, which spared the pain of the classroom but gained condemnation instead. Had I had the opportunity to grope toward what I sensed I needed, I might have found it, but there were no alternatives for children then.

Sometimes I conformed, went to school and suffered; sometimes I rebelled, refused, and suffered.

---

[*] This article first appeared in *Women Look at Psychiatry*, Dorothy E. Smith and Sara J. David, eds. (Vancouver, BC: Press Gang Publishers, 1975).

Adolescence added the further torment of sex. In the repressive late 1950s, a time of rigidly stereotyped gender roles, I both longed for and feared the attentions of boys, who were strangers, almost aliens. Once again, it seemed that any choice was only a choice of which pain I was to suffer.

My parents, only dimly sensing my agony (we did not speak of such things to one another), sent me to a psychiatrist. It seemed logical to them, loving me and wanting to ease my pain. It seemed logical to me as well: out of step for so many years, I now had powerful confirmation that the fault lay within me.

The choices were so limited: continuing my education—voluntarily once high school was agonizingly completed, a job (and what kind of a job for a woman—without a degree, with no training or experience) or salvation through love (and what an easy conclusion for a child of the 1950s).

In 1965, I married. Redemption, so I thought, through the roles of wife and mother—at last, no longer out of step. In a few months I was pregnant, radiant, joyous, at last successful in a role. Then miscarriage—failure!—and collapse.

Again I encounter a psychiatrist, this time a dispenser of magic pills. I went to his office, cried, was given a handful of multicolored goodies, went home, cried, and swallowed pills. He was puzzled that I was not "improving." He suggested hospitalization. Out of longing to end the pain (pain I could not understand, for hadn't I—for once—done everything *right*?), I agreed.

In March 1966, I signed myself into the psychiatric ward of Mt. Sinai Hospital, seeking warmth, support, and psychotherapy. The hospital's first act was to change my medication. Then, disoriented as well as depressed, I moved through the hospital's program of occupational and recreational "therapy." The first lesson to the mental patient, repeated in varying forms in every hospital I was ever in was clear: Behave! Conform! Never directly stated, the message was nevertheless all too clear. The lesson of the first 21 years of my life was thus repeated, this time by an institution of force, since I had failed to learn the lesson as taught by more benevolent institutions.

I had entered the hospital in an attempt to find relief for the pain of living, and found, instead, that any attempt to show this pain to my "healers," so they could understand and help me, was swiftly met with repression. A good patient was one who swallowed the medication, followed the hospital routine, and indicated a willingness to "cope" with the life circumstances that had brought about hospitalization in the first place. Breaking out of the prison, "rebelling," was a symptom of one's illness. Conformity was mental health.

Discharged after two-and-a-half weeks, I went home to my prison. There was no women's movement to help me see that my cold and unrewarding marriage was a trap; I became convinced that since I saw it as a prison, I was still "crazy." So I tried to convince myself that I was lucky (didn't I have a "good" husband, a "nice" apartment?), and continued to cry.

The lesson was still unlearned. Despite all the authority figures who had failed in the past to entrust me with the secret of life (which I still believed they held and could somehow be persuaded to part with), I now decided psychiatrists were the ones with the mystical "answer." Nothing in my experience had given me the confidence to seek it within myself, the lonely, the out-of-step, the sick one. I returned to the hospital, desperate to be "helped." They had "no room," turned me away, sent me in a police ambulance to Bellevue. Bellevue—childhood taunt, nightmare of the unknown, cold shiver in the dark. Was it once a hill, overlooking a beautiful expanse of water? An estate, perhaps, with children playing on the lawn? Ugly buildings, crumbling yet still strong, thick walls—but the name suggests that perhaps there was a time before the ugliness. I never saw it clearly; first, they took away my glasses.

Half-blind, I groped along the hallway to my bed, pointed out to me by a bored aide. I wanted her to lead me to it—I was afraid of falling or stumbling—but she only waved. It was night, beds everywhere, snores and moans. I tried to get up for a drink of water and was yelled back to bed.

My parents, horrified, made inquiries, pulled strings with money they didn't have and had me transferred to Gracie Square Hospital, a place where rich alcoholics dried out and rich psychotics were zapped at $50 a shock. Terrified, having seen the price for disobedience (for I had defied the psychiatrists by not resuming my role), I tried hard now to be "good." The carpeted floors and pastel walls showed me one of my choices; the vacant stares and shuffling gaits of the patients returning each morning from the shock room showed the other. Again, the lesson: conformity or punishment!

▲ ▲ ▲

Why was I so convinced there was some secret, if only I could persuade them to share it with me, that I was led continually back to the hospital and closer to danger? I watched, uncomprehending, how "normal" people moved without effort through the routines that seemed to me so deadly and stifling, and I was sure there *must* be a secret, that *they* shared and from which *I* was excluded. Again and again, I risked the punishment of drugs, the threats of shock and continued confinement, desperate to find a way to continue to live. In the meaningless rituals of life, I saw only death. *And I wanted to live.*

I know now that my terror had a very real basis—it was not "crazy" after all, but a confirmation of my sanity. The rituals were meaningless, such "life" was truly death. Having moved all my life from role to role—sometimes being dragged, sometimes all too willingly—I was making a desperate attempt to truly live for the first time. I was struggling to be born. And struggling alone—I was being forced toward death rather than life.

Convinced of my weakness, wrongness, and craziness, I could not believe that the answer lay within me. No one was trying to tell me of my strength: calling me crazy was confirmation that I was weak and powerless. If someone had been there saying, "Yes, go on, feel it, see it through to the end," my life story might have been very different.

I left the shock shop unshocked. How incredibly lucky I was! Patient in six hospitals, suffering from "depression"—the prime "indication" for shock—then labeled with the stigmatizing diagnosis of catatonic or chronic schizophrenia, and never "treated" with the wires and switches of ECT! How did I escape?

Terror had me truly immobilized. A move in any direction seemed certain to bring death or destruction. Should I start "functioning" again in a marriage in which I already defined myself as a failure? Leave it and go back to—what? Follow the vague stirrings of a mind I had been convinced was crazy? The only way to stay alive was to do nothing.

I turned again to the wisdom of my psychiatrist. Surely, somewhere, he had the answer. If only I would be good (but it didn't seem I was ever good enough), he would reveal to me the secret of life, the secret of normality. The next psychiatric "treatment" for me was the structured environment: a hospital where every moment of the patient's day was regulated with "therapeutic" purpose. It sounded like a way of staying alive.

But Hillside Hospital was a farce. Unknowing or uncaring of my fear of the death I thought was imminent, the staff processed me through its routine. The "structured environment" prescribed that I could make no phone calls and see no visitors until I "earned" those privileges, that I could not step out of my "cottage" without a staff member, that I must participate in the daily program that combined the worst features of school and summer camp. The fact that all these requirements and prohibitions terrified me concerned no one: it was something I must do; it was my therapy. I was facing the terror of my own death, and they wanted me to mold clay. I was taken into an expensively equipped woodworking shop and asked to guide a board past a moving saw—I screamed and fled in terror of slicing off an arm—I was uncooperative.

After this incident, I became desperate to leave the place I had been so eager to enter. The entrance procedure had been as complex and harrowing as a college admission. My action had been toward life; instead, it seemed they were trying to crush the last bits of life in me. I used every means I could think of to convince them to let me leave: screams, tears, punches, logical argument. They could easily have "shipped" me. ("Shipped" was hospital slang for being committed to a state hospital.) Instead, they released me.

I was out in the dangerous world again. I slit my wrists. I entered the psychiatric ward of Montefiore Hospital. I was trying to stay alive.

I needed time, safety, and support. For a while, I was given the time and the safety. I began to breathe a little more easily, feeling that perhaps my death was not imminent after all. But psychiatry is never content to do nothing, to let time be the healer. I was put on tranquilizers again. I protested, argued, begged, and finally resorted to hiding the pills in my mouth and spitting them in the toilet. Uncooperative again. My safe place was no longer safe; I knew that drugs bent my mind and increased the feeling that something awful was about to happen. I begged to be released and was told, "No, you're too sick." I longed for some place safe, quiet, warm, where I could grow whole again. Suddenly, doors that had been opened were locked; I was forbidden to go outside, even escorted. Panic—I knew that unless I found the mythical "safe place" I would die. Panic—I pounded at the locked door and screamed my desperation.

Uncooperative patients are punished. I was committed to Rockland State Hospital.

The lesson finally learned. Freedom was an illusion. Only cooperation brought life. That life seemed like a living death was a cruel joke. But it was better than the punishment of confinement and depersonalization. I promised to be "good." There was no escape.

But first I had to be sent to the state hospital, bear the indignities to mind and body, prove that I was truly docile, broken, "cured." Only then could I be set free, confirmed in the belief that to walk endlessly through the motions of a living death was truly life, happiness and health.

It would be years before I would once again risk the struggle of being born.

AFTERWORD

"Struggling to be Born" describes a period in my life when I was virtually without hope. Things were not to change for me for many years; one of the major factors in that change for me was becoming part of the mental patients' liberation movement. For more than twenty years, working within a number of groups composed of former patients, I have been able to forge a new and far more satisfying life. What I only dimly perceived during the period described in "Struggling to be Born," and what the psychiatric system did its best to obscure, is that there is truth in our madness. We are told that we are defective human beings and that we need hospitalization and drugs to control the disorder. Each of us, isolated and alone, has little choice but to believe these myths. It is only when we join together, when we tell each other our stories, that we begin to see another reality: that each of us "goes crazy" for a reason, and that we must change our lives rather than our brain chemistry.

What is now usually called the psychiatric survivor movement is an effort to bring about change both on the political level, so that we may no longer be locked up and drugged against our will, and on the personal level, so that each of us, when we are suffering, can turn to our peers for comfort. We are a long way from achieving that goal, but thousands of people around the world are part of that effort. I am proud to be one of them.

HOSPITAL RECORDS

Jeanine Grobe

I don't know why I want my hospital records—after so many years, why now?—but I do. The first step is to call and ask for them.

"It is against hospital policy to release a patient's records to the patient," I am told.

"Why?" I ask.

"Patients misinterpret things. These records are for professionals."

Patients? I'm not a patient, I'm a former patient. They signed the discharge papers. I'm not supposed to "misinterpret" things anymore.

Stay calm, I tell myself, like a good mental patient.

I know enough about psychiatric "medicine" to interpret any psychiatric hospital record, but clearly, this is not the issue. The issue is *power*.

My next question is about this hospital policy and my rights as a former psychiatric patient. Clearly, the person I'm speaking with at the hospital has more important things to do than talk to me. I am becoming a real bother and, besides, she can't answer my question. She'll have to connect me with someone "higher up," but first she asks me, "Is this really that important to you?" and second, "Haven't you been feeling well?" In other words, wanting a copy of my hospital records is interpreted as a sign of illness.

Finally, I reach the higher up connection. He tells me exactly the same thing the first person did—verbatim. The person he connects me to tells me the same, and, finally, the person I *should* talk to is not in.

My next step is to contact the attorney advocate. He informs me, without doubt, that access to the records is my legal right. He dictates a letter over the phone for me to send to the psychiatric hospital requesting my records.

Good, it's finally moving.

I receive a letter in response: "It is against hospital policy to release records . . . blah blah blah."

I call the attorney advocate again. "How do they think they can get away with this?" he says. Sensing my doubt, he sends me a photocopy of the law. I sign a consent form accompanying *his* request to obtain the records. In a few weeks I pick the records up at his office, and the real fun begins.

▲ ▲ ▲

I sit in my car holding the thick envelope. One small victory in my hands. I hadn't given in, let them intimidate me, stop me. I open the envelope. I see the photocopy print, in a square at the top:

> Principal Diagnosis: Brief Reactive Psychosis.
> Date of admission: September 25, 1988.

Yes. My last hospitalization. I remember. I remember it well.

With all of the problems I have had, a poor memory has never been among them. Quite the opposite. I graduated college summa cum laude, often breaking instructors' grading curves. Because I'm so smart? I wish. No, it's my memory. It's very good. I remember my last hospitalization.

I continue reading:

> The patient lives with her parents in Lakeville.

This is wrong. My parents never lived in Lakeville; I lived there alone. So what, who cares. Then I read:

> The patient was suicidal and homicidal at the start of
> hospitalization.

What? I read this again. I check the top line to make sure it is *my* name on the record. I remember not sleeping, not eating, and nightmares. I remember the inability to form sentences, to create meaning, to communicate. I remember feeling horrified.

But suicidal? Homicidal? No. I've never been homicidal. Suicidal, yes. But not this time.

These "records" are pure fabrication. But why?

I remember the call to my friend: "Cathy, please don't let them commit me."

I hand the phone to the admitting physician and hear Cathy's voice emphatically over the phone: "I am her therapist and I do not want her in there."

The physician is unruffled. "We disagree," he says.

I look at the skull and crossbones labeling the telephone dial. Appropriate.

He hands the phone back to me.

"We'll get you out of there," Cathy says.

Her last words to me were, "Don't even give them your tears."

The next day my mother came. She threatened to call a lawyer.

The physician laughed, "You won't get anywhere, we have our own."

As he exited, she called to him, "Are you above God too?"

▲ ▲ ▲

They had no grounds to commit me, even by their own standards, but they did it. Against my will, against my "therapist's" will, against my parents' will. So they cover themselves: "Suicidal. Homicidal." And cover themselves:

> The patient appeared to be responding to auditory hallucinations at the time of admission. She denied this was so, but she was clearly seen by several staff members talking to others and responding to such.

Auditory hallucinations. The tell-tale sign of "psychosis," the mark of SERIOUS psychiatric disorder. Good cover.

They could tell I was having them, though I denied and still deny it. I must conclude: They could hear through my ears—and heard things I didn't. Not that I've never experienced hallucinations. I have, following the administration of antipsychotic drugs. Here's what they have to say about that:

The patient was treated with various antipsychotic
medications and lithium in previous hospitalizations. She
has a history of being noncompliant with medication use.

Noncompliant? Oh dear. I guess I should WANT to
hallucinate.

▲ ▲ ▲

I finally reach the end of the first discharge summary:

The patient responded quickly to the supportive milieu
within the environment of the hospital over the course of
48 hours.

Successful treatment of homicidal, suicidal, "psychotic"
woman in 48 hours. Wow. They should advertise this.

And about responding "quickly to the supportive milieu
within the environment of the hospital," I'm laughing, sort of.
I hid in my room for 48 hours so they couldn't use the fear in
my eyes, fear of being there, as a reason to keep me there. They
claim it as their victory.

Lest I forget the omissions, of which there are too many,
here's one: they forgot to record what happened to the five
dollars that was in my bag. But, that's right, I was "disorganized
and confused." They're covered.

My conclusion about hospital policy for staff members:

▲ When they don't know, they make it up.
▲ When they do know, they still make it up.

I'm exhausted now and put the records aside. I drive home
wondering whether I should read the rest. Is it worth the
aggravation? The frustration of seeing lies recorded about me
on legal files? Maybe this one is an exception.

I finish reading the records, in small doses, over the next few
days. No exception.

Comic relief is provided only by some of the more
inconsequential inaccuracies:

The patient is 4'11".

I'm 5'2".

a psychology student

Close: music and philosophy.
The rest gives me a belly ache and I wonder, after so many years, how I survived it:

Patient's condition improved with neuroleptics.

I recall a mental health worker who was becoming increasingly skeptical about the whole psychiatric business. While I was sitting with a cup of coffee, trying to revive myself after an injection that caused unconsciousness for nearly 24 hours, he pulled up a chair beside me and remarked on the "absurdity" of what goes on at these places: "for instance, they overdose a patient and on the report you read, 'patient's condition improved.'"

Out of the corner of his mouth came my link to the real world.

Chemotherapy is not the only absurdity. The "quiet room" shares the stage:

After time in the quiet room, the patient was more cooperative.

I recall the first time I was put in seclusion. Five large men were standing around me, all ninety pounds of me, ready to give me an escort to the "quiet room." (I'd been protesting too loudly.)

"I'll move myself," I told them, frightened, obliging, "please let me."

But they lifted me into the air and carried me anyway.

I'd never been locked into a room I couldn't get out of. I developed claustrophobia instantly. Hours later, I walked out a different woman.

The next day, a patient was refusing her medication. I knew what they'd do to her if she continued, so I tried to warn her: "They'll put you in there!" I pointed to the room.

The nurse looked at me, satisfied. "You learned your lesson," she admonished me.

She thought I thought I was in a mental hospital.
I thought I was in hell.

▲ ▲ ▲

I never said anything about the mental health worker who, after accidentally opening the door on a young woman showering, continued to watch for several minutes. Nor did I say anything about that same mental health worker when he fondled my breasts after "catching" me in an attempt to "elope" from the hospital. So these incidents do not appear in the records.

But the verbal cruelty of one night worker caused me so much distress that I lived in dread of the evenings he worked. I did report him. And it appears in the records:

> The patient made an attempt to split staff members.

▲ ▲ ▲

Rights of a mental patient?

> She exhibits a thought disorder including a belief in transcendental phenomenon and other bizarre ideation of her own personal socioreligious philosophy.

So much for the First Amendment.

▲ ▲ ▲

How about this one:

> The patient was apparently raped at age 15. She has a history of sexual promiscuity.

In order to feel the full impact of this, you have to know something about me. At the age of 37, I have had exactly two serious "romantic" relationships and seven or eight isolated dates. I am not passing judgment on promiscuous behavior here but on the fact that the statement is untrue, and then, of course, on the fact that appearing as it does after the statement that I was "apparently" raped suggests that I was somehow responsible for the rape.

I had read this particular record a few months after my first hospitalization 16 years ago when my former psychiatrist obtained a copy and allowed me to read it. When confronted by my puzzlement, he coolly explained—well, you know how it is, someone misinterprets something, something is misunderstood, it gets recorded wrong, there's confusion—you know how it is.

Yeah, aren't I lucky?

▲ ▲ ▲

As I turn through the pages of these records, I am struck by the fact that I can barely get past two lines without finding something objectionable. In conclusion, I'd be tempted to say that these records are bullshit except that bullshit rots and eventually feeds the earth. These records are not rotting; they are kept very much alive by the legal system which honors them and the psychiatric institutions that continue to produce others like them.

▲ ▲ ▲

"Mental illness." The words were always meaningless to me.

"You have to understand, you have an illness," the doctors would say.

The way I experience life, myself, the world is an illness. My perceptions, sensations, thoughts, feelings, memories, my dreams. All illness.

"What exactly is this illness?" I asked a doctor once.

"We really don't know," he answered.

When I insisted that I needed some kind of perspective, some framework, he studied me for a moment, then informed me that he was increasing the dosage on my Thorazine because "these feelings of meaninglessness can become quite a problem."

Yes. Meaninglessness can be a problem. He should know.

▲ ▲ ▲

About a year after this conversation, I met a shaman/healer. This woman met my pain and confusion with stories, stories that provided a framework for my experiences, a point of relation that allowed me to embrace the process of my own being in the world.

She didn't reduce my pain to some brain abnormality. She simply made it meaningful.

People have asked me what made this person succeed where the "professionals" failed. The answer to that is *experience*.

What was different about my shaman friend was that she had no fear of "madness." She had experienced many varieties of consciousness in herself and knew the territory well. She was a seasoned traveller in the very places psychiatry is afraid of, in the places it claims to understand but has no experience of, in the places it prescribes "treatment" to avoid.

▲ ▲ ▲

The mental health system has kept records on me for 17 years. The last one was made in September 1988. This is my first record on them.

JUNGLE DREAMING

Beth Greenspan

JUNGLE DREAMING—JUNGLE DREAMING
Swinging on vines of the wild world
Breaking loose from the hurting stiffness of buildings
Tied down medicated tree climbing—JUNGLE
    DREAMING—
JUNGLE DREAMING I'm fourteen floors up concretely
    swaying
In the heavy-eyed, fake-aired atmosphere
With cautiously smiling nurses and you are under me
Somewhere surviving the bells that will ring at
    twelve-thirty
I will be automatically looking for food and coffee
Looking for the doctor who whispers in back rooms
Monitors the transformations tranquilizations
And they don't need a dart gun they've got
Pretty faces instead with soft dark eyes
To administer the ends of worlds—JUNGLE
    DREAMING
I am dreaming in my jungle bed of twisted vine sheets
Low hum of Afrikan waters trickling in these ancient
Dark suffering vein walls engraved with air conditioners
Carved with sagas of madness in dead winter
Meetings over empty tables a car honking down on 11th
    street—
JUNGLE DREAMING—nobody thinks of you and me
    slipping away
Below us floors of Xerox machines to copy what they've
Written about us or what we have to say soon to be buried

In the basement of this tomb—vitals and all we are
    rotting—JUNGLE DREAMING—I've had enough
Prayer—silence—door slams.

SURVIVOR PRIDE

Catherine Odette

I am a person living with a psychiatric disability. I have pride in who I am. I have pride in being a person with a psychiatric disability.

The current treatment for a person with a psychiatric disability is hospitalization—including all its sub-"treatments," like drugs, time in seclusion, time in four-point restraint. I almost didn't survive the treatment for my disability. My psychiatric disability is tough enough to live with—but the treatments almost killed me!

For almost 15 years, I lived in state hospitals, receiving treatment for my psychiatric disability. I received drugs as part of my treatment. The levels of Thorazine and Stelazine I was taking are now considered toxic, even by some of the most conservative prescribing physicians. My mind was a toxic dump. I was chemically straitjacketed, almost incapable of thought. Often, because I tried to refuse these drugs, they were forced into my body. I knew, even in the nearly unconscious state of my toxic wasteland that those drugs were wrong and were damaging me.

Electroconvulsive shock was another part of my "treatment." My spine would take that classic unnatural arc during the count: One-one thousand, two-one thousand, three-one thousand, four-one thousand. The seizures shattered most of my teeth. Sixty electric shock treatments later, that treatment was discontinued. I guess it didn't work the way the professionals thought it might. Now they use anesthesia to prevent the breaking bones and teeth.

The next two treatments, restraint and seclusion, were often combined. I was locked in a room. This room had no bed, only

75

a mattress on the floor. No lamp for bedtime reading. No pitcher of ice water in case I was thirsty. No scenes of pastoral beauty graced the walls. No radio eased my transition to sleep. No chamber pot, no commode, no private bath off the bedroom. No place to wash, no place to toilet. No privacy, no heat, no safety.

I was forced to live in that room as part of my treatment. I was forced to use the floor of that room as my toilet. I broke windows to let out the stench and was left to enjoy a winter in seclusion. The mattress that was my bed was often used by the staff to smother me against the wall, while an injection was forced into my arm or buttocks. When extra treatment was needed, a metal bed was brought in so that there was someplace to tie the leather restraints, wrist and ankle, usually face down. My food came to me on a tray, usually without utensils. As often as not, it was slid across the room to me—gliding on my own urine!

Nighttime is always a special thing in a mental hospital. The noisy rest of the other residents is almost indescribable. People cry out for help in their sleep. People fight against the leather cuffs of restraint. People sleep with protection. A fork is a prized possession on the wards. When HE comes to your bed, that mammoth key ring jangling with each step, a fork is a good thing to have.

You don't get forks in seclusion. You can't get to your fork if you are tied by the ankle and by the wrist, sometimes a strap across your throat or forehead. You can't defend yourself against the staffman who decides you're IT. You can't defend yourself against the memories of witnessing the rape of your roommate. There's almost nothing you can tell yourself to stop the memory of witnessing the rape of your roommate.

▲ ▲ ▲

Pride in my psychiatric disability didn't come easily. Pride came with my job, my political activism, and recovery from the abuse offered as treatment in state hospitals.

Those treatments, restraint and seclusion, did not cure my psychiatric disability. Neither restraint nor seclusion will ever cure a psychiatric disability. They are inhumane. They set the stage for sexual abuse. They degrade and damage people, causing their own set of trauma reactions. They escalate anger and so-called acting-out behavior. They don't work! They are wrong! They should be illegal!

Today, I have what everyone always said they wanted me to have . . . a life! That means I have a full-time job. I have friends. I have a life-partner and together we have a home, complete with a cat and dishes in the sink. I do volunteer work, I am politically active, and I have a reputation of which I am proud. I have my dignity. I have my pride. I have my self. I, alone, make choices about every aspect of my life. I, alone, make all decisions that affect my life.

I also have the scars that serve to remind me of times when decisions about my life were not my own. Those were times when the DMH found this human being, who is me, invisible. They had me. Their actions say they wanted to kill me, and so, they had me by the wrists, by the ankles, by the hours, by the weeks, by my reputation, by my pride, by my dignity.

Today, I have my heart, each beat emptying and refilling the chambers with those memories that refuse to be quieted or replaced. I remember seclusion. I remember restraint.

Today, I have my teeth, mostly shattered, mostly ruined. One-one thousand, two-one thousand, three-one thousand, four-one thousand. I remember not remembering. I remember nothingness after the shock treatments.

Today, I have my wrist scars. I have the thick white lines, indicating not a place for the wrist to fold, but the place where I folded, where I could no longer bear my imprisonment.

Today I have my mind, where an internal movie without end flashes vivid, lightning images of a single room from the state hospital. That room of my imprisonment, that room where I lived in my own excrement. That room where I was made available to the unwanted, the truly sick "affections"—where, because I was imprisoned by drugs and leather-cuff restraint, I was subject to the sexual aberrations of key-holding attendants.

The Department of Mental Health (DMH) may want to claim success for my functioning in spite of my serious mental illness. They may want to flaunt me, "See what we did for this patient?" THEY HAD BETTER NOT DARE to claim any measure of this woman's health. I survived in spite of the DMH, and I bear all the scars and memories of my imprisonment.

I was invisible when I was a patient; when the treatment for my mental illness broke my body, my health, my spirit. The act of speaking from the living pages of this book makes me visible.

I want to be seen. I want *you* to dare to see the human being. I want you to dare to acknowledge the depth of stigma you impose on me. I dare you to see the scars of your "treatments." I dare you to put shackles on your very own children who are "out of control" or who are "acting out." If you are shocked, if your own soul rebels against this idea, then you have made a dent in the illogic so often applied to people within DMH custody.

A DAY IN THE LIFE OF LARRY THE PLANT*

Angie Hopkins Hart

I have seen so many people come and go over the years; it makes me weary to know that no one has ever bothered to tend or nurture me. And now I need repotting urgently. My leaves are so yellow and brown that I am dying.

I would like to relate to you the lives and turmoils I have witnessed from this particular spot in the middle of this particular coffeetable—my vantagepoint set against a nicotine-stained wall. I am in what is called a day room in a hospital. Not just an ordinary hospital; one of the biggest hospitals in Europe, in England, the land of green and plenty. Allow me to get inside your mind and take you on a journey.

Chapter One

"I wonder what's for breakfast," said Lacey to Cagney. They're the two goldfish swimming in the tank on the other side of the room from me.

"Same as yesterday," said Cagney. "What's up with you? We get fish flakes 365 days a year—and you're wondering what's for breakfast? Have you gone a bit batty like all these puddled people around us!"

Lacey replies, "Well, they get a choice. Fish fingers on Monday (it makes me paranoid when they have fish fingers),

---

* This is an excerpt from *Sally the Sane Schizophrenic*, a book in progress.

scrambled egg on Tuesday, beans or spaghetti Wednesday and Thursday, and sausages on Friday. Plus a choice of mueseli or porridge and a cup of tea. I'm sick of getting fish flakes 365 days a year. I want a cup of tea."

On overhearing this conversation coming from the fish tank, I knew Lacey was getting on in years.

In fact, she's been here nearly as long as I have. And I know how Lacey felt. Sick as a parrot. (Good job we didn't have a parrot as well.) Sick to the back teeth. Suffering from senility. Dropping dead from old age.

I looked around me just in time to see a new patient arrive. Oh dear. What a state.

In the meantime, the chef has been on a stag-night. He is getting married on Saturday. It is now Friday morning, and Thursday evening has just passed with great exhilaration—a pub crawl. The deputy chef was with him buying pint after pint, vodka after vodka. In the end, they'd become oblivious. They got taken to Casualty and were both admitted with alcohol poisoning. Thus, they were unable to go to work, cooking breakfasts on the wing for all these psychiatric patients. Furthermore, when these two particularly inebriated chefs awoke, they couldn't remember who they were, let alone that they were supposed to be cooking breakfast for seven wards and 215 people. So nobody had any breakfast, except Cagney and Lacey whose routine wasn't disrupted, and they got fed fish flakes as usual.

Chapter Two

Oh dear, another long day ahead. I wonder what's happening in the dormitories. Sally was very pleased to get a bed next to the radiator and sink, so she could be warm and could make sure no one nicks her toothpaste.

But she doesn't look too happy this morning. If I could speak, I would have warned her that she was in the bed next to Rita, a compulsive handwasher. Sally's been kept awake all night by the taps going on and off. Poor lass.

Chapter Three

Who else is here? Nobody—there doesn't seem to be anybody else here. That's unusual. I suppose it's like the lull in a supermarket when you and your fellow plants are waiting to be bought. Sometimes you don't lose anybody, and other times you lose three of four friends in a day.

As soon as someone starts buying, someone else comes along and copies them. It must be the same with this so called "mental illness." Once one person gets it, there's a queue of jealous people wanting it as well.

I don't know why. Having spent the past ten years of my life rooted to this spot observing bizarre behavior, I don't know why anyone would want it. I don't suppose they choose to get it, it just happens to them.

They find themselves being able to hear the voices that I beam into their minds with my telepathic rays. Or they find themselves ripping up newspapers or novels. Or sometimes the poor dears are fed-up. Sometimes they have lost a loved one. Suffered unrequited love. Or society just won't accept them the way they are and this is where they end up.

I wouldn't wish it on my worst enemy, even Colin the Cactus who kept pricking me on the supermarket shelf. He's in Scotland now. But he warned me—it could happen to you.

Chapter Four

A nurse suddenly sees the patient, Sally, heading for the door and shouts out, "Sally, where are you going?"

Sally replies, "I'm going for a walk."

The nurse is pleased to see Sally taking an interest in the "outside world"; normally Sally's too paranoid to go off the ward.

"But don't you think people will stare at you?" the nurse inquires politely.

"No," Sally states simply. "It's too foggy."

Oh well, Sally's not made a miraculous recovery after all but found a simple cure to stop people from looking at her—fog. Nobody can see a darn thing.

Chapter Five

We are all sitting around watching television when suddenly Sally jumps up and yells out, "What a word to write to life living in total darkness, no way to walk amongst these winding streets."

A sudden pang of angst stabs my very soul as I wonder if Sally has twigged that I, Larry the Plant, am writing about her.

Fortunately, one of the nurses responds to her, "Sally, sit down and be quiet please, people are trying to watch television." A salve for my guilty conscience. I'm sure she wouldn't mind me writing about her anyway. Maybe I will ask her. I send her a voice that the nurses and doctors cannot hear, "Sally, do you mind me writing about you?"

Sally leaps up again. This time it's not because of the side-effects of Largactil but because she has heard a voice—my voice.

She yells out, "What are your words writhing below ground level aimed at?" Sally can get quite incoherent but I still get her meaning. She wants to know what I'm writing about. The nurse just thinks she's paranoid.

The nurse responds firmly, "Sally, what's the matter, oh dear, come with me and I'll give you something to help these funny thoughts of yours."

Sally gets upset and yells, "But I don't like Largactil, I don't like Largactil, I don't like Largactil!"

"Come on, you're too upset to stay in the day room, take this medicine and go to bed," the nurse tells her.

I just put my dying flowers on my dying leaves in despair. I've got the poor lass in trouble again.

Chapter Six

In this strange universe called Ward 11, there's nothing left to say. Time revolves differently here. Time has stopped altogether for some people. I don't know what Cagney and Lacey think about it all. I don't want to interrupt them while they're having a cozy chat round the back of the ornamental arch next to the air bubbler. I see tails waggling eagerly but that's about it.

I wonder. MMMnnnn. We plants do that but we never get any fun apart from a passing honey bee rubbing against our stamen and you don't get any honey bees in here. Oh oh, Cagney's run off and Lacey's chasing her. Stevie, the right-on feminist and morning domestic on this ward has gone to see what they're up to. As if it isn't obvious.

"Have a good peek, Stevie," I beam telepathically into his mind. Unfortunately, he can't hear me. He's not schizophrenic like Sally. Sally's really intelligent. Stevie's intelligent too, he just uses it in a different way. He's never had any traumas in his life.

I'd tell you about Stevie and his many ways of making Sally's life a misery, but I don't want to sound bitter. It's none of my business really.

Chapter Seven— The Final Chapter

Sally's mum comes to visit Sally. She doesn't like the way the hospital is run, the way the patients are left to sit in the day room all day long staring at a mindless TV set. I don't like the way these poor people are treated either. If only I could find a way out. A solution to my and Sally's problems.

Now take Sally's mum. A fine person. A good, strong determined woman. A friendly face. An understanding way of speaking. I wonder. "Mum, please take me home with you," Sally asks her mother.

Poor Sally's mum is tortured. She scarcely knows what to do for the best. Could she really look after Sally at home? After all, she doesn't like leaving her here, but how is she to go to work every day? And what can Sally do all day long? Maybe Sally could go to a day center during the day.

"I can't, really love. I'm working all day long," Sally's mum responds.

"Mum, please take me home with you," Sally pleads.

Sally doesn't understand why she's in this strange place not at all like her family's home and wonders why she's not allowed to go to work. She misses her job and her boyfriend (who's deserted her). All her routine has been disrupted and she can't understand why. I can see she wants out. So do I. I never get watered either.

"Mum, please take me home with you," Sally cries again.

This final plea left Sally's mum relenting. She was heartbroken at leaving her daughter here in this forlorn forgotten institution. She'd love to have Sally home as she misses her dreadfully.

She gave in, "All right Sally, I'll take you home."

I couldn't believe it. Sally was leaving me. I suddenly panicked and screamed out wildly, "Take me with you!" I didn't want to die here.

Sally looked up in surprise, and as she did, she noticed me and my brown withered, dying leaves shrieking in agony. Quickly, she picked me up and Sally's mum took hold of Sally's hand and led her out to the car. Sally held me carefully, gently, and I knew that she and her kind and warm-natured mum would see me right. I resolved not to use my telepathic rays to beam any more voices into Sally's brain.

At home Sally recovered, and so did I, but did we all live happily ever after?

THE 13th STATE*

Batya Weinbaum

1

She was sleeping with men again in order to kill time. She looked at it as activity therapy, as they say in the hospital. She had begun to pick up men in the streets in New York when it all began—how long ago. She had lost track of time. If she killed enough time, she thought, she would distract herself from killing herself.

She couldn't see into the future, into the end. One man after another, sometimes two or three in a week. The roommates would put her out soon, she suspected. Who knew if it would be the men, or all the letters from social services she had to get them to sign, that finally drove them to it.

She played cards and chess with the men. Sometimes they took her to plays and to movies. Sometimes they fed her; sometimes she fed them. The one with white hair always wanted to buy her sweets; one a silk bathrobe; one gave her money for vitamins. One taught her to sing.

She had fallen in love with the psychiatrist at the hospital. No one else had ever seemed so good. She had gone back four times, she knew, in order to be with him. He cared about her, he had said. And no one else could make her feel so good. She had become hooked on the embraces, the conversations. She was

---

* The following is a fictionalized account. Any resemblance to actual persons or places is purely coincidental. It first appeared in a slightly different form in *Phoenix Rising*, vol 2, no 3, 1981.

a wild woman, the white-haired one said. She had magic and charm, said the others.

She knew she could never outlive the memories. Jumping the fence at the hospital, hitchhiking. The truck drivers on the CB getting rides for the beaver. The one in Massachusetts she had been going to meet, who wanted to save her with ideas about Jesus. The drug dealer in the park saying, have you tried a black man, selling her black beauties. The palm reader saying she'd be dead by the end of the year.

She was mentally ill and she knew it. The shrinks knew it. The people she used to know stopped knowing her. She couldn't go back to her parents. They'd put her in the hospital again. She would run around screaming at everyone again or withdraw into her room doing nothing but pulling out her hair and squeezing her nipples. Or perhaps she would develop the control and stop speaking, just write little notes on pink and yellow notecards to everyone: DON'T SAY ANYTHING TO ME, PLEASE. I WANT MY PRIVACY, MY BOUNDARIES. YOU WON'T SAY ANYTHING I HAVEN'T HEARD BEFORE. I AM NOT BEING HOSTILE. I DON'T WANT TO SCREAM AT YOU. JUST, I HAVE TROUBLE DEVELOPING EGO DEFENSES AND THIS IS MY FIRST ONE. KINDLY, LEAVE ME. . . .

Or little stamps, like at the stationery store, which she could sit in her room and stamp hard all over her blank paper, or again on little cards: BE PASSIVE AND OBEDIENT. SHUT UP AND DO WHAT YOU'RE TOLD. DON'T TRUST SHRINKS, EVER AGAIN. I HATE MY MOTHER I HATE MY FATHER I HATE MYSELF.

Last time, she had thrown shoes one at a time against the wall, screaming at the thud of each one:

> I am a DRAIN
> I am a BURDEN
> and I CAUSE PAIN
> I am a DRAIN
> I am a BURDEN
> and I CAUSE PAIN
> I am a DRAIN
> I am a BURDEN
> and I CAUSE PAIN . . .

She had just gotten into the staccato rhythm, experiencing some relief, some discharge, some lift of the externalized violence, venting her anger on the wall rather than inwardly upon herself, when the nurses had entered, to check out her "anti-social behavior" which, since she had been told she had, she had developed, steadfastly. . . . The red-haired nurse had taken charge and overruled the orders of the doctor to give her her clothes and take her out for a walk. She had been locked up in isolation for two weeks, without her glasses, without her clothes, without her notecards . . . no rights, no activities, no passes.

That was the past. The scene she had run away from, with her father on the phone later cursing her: "You knew what I wanted you to do." How could she scream at him a line she had learned from previous therapy, IF CHILDREN DID WHAT THEIR PARENTS WANTED THERE WOULD BE NO PROGRESS IN CIVILIZATION . . . THAT'S WHY I RAN . . . CAN'T YOU UNDERSTAND ME. . . .

▲ ▲ ▲

There she was, broke and starving in New York, feeling like an urchin. She had dreams about the psychiatrist coming to make love to her, if she lived in a cheap, lower east side, crummy apartment. Or of the excitement of the whistle blowing, all the patients hustling down the mountain like at summer camp, to tuck into their bunk beds for the emergency whistle, the fun, the excitement, something going on, very important, and all the patients were needed apparently. How fun to see everyone! And immediately she had hugged and apologized to the doctor. He had smiled at her.

She burst into tears at the slightest provocation, feeling as vulnerable on the streets of New York as she had in the hospital. The one who was teaching her to sing—she had sung for a while and withdrawn again. She couldn't talk, she couldn't explain it really. He said she didn't have to talk, and she tried to use the advice the psychiatrists gave her: don't be so open. It all flashed through her mind so quickly. Here he was teaching her to sing, this one. Activity therapy. And she had gotten despairing about all the things people had tried to do for her, which all seemed like pulling her off center, off herself.

The psychiatrists couldn't understand it, her parents couldn't, her brother couldn't. But it felt like being pulled off, she felt evaporated, she felt as if she disappeared into whatever people projected onto her. The psychiatrist thought she should marry a doctor (where would she meet a nice 29-year-old Jewish physician, someone of the same background, he had asked her), go into the helping professions, help other people. How could she explain how she identified with the needy and felt needier. The Mexican murderer she met at the Plaza. He wouldn't do her in. She called every week asking if he had gotten the pills. He kept saying no, survival was hard for everyone, the pusher wasn't on the streets, try again.

▲ ▲ ▲

*Sometimes I feel like a black animal cringing in the forest waiting for some prince charming to come along and tap me on the head with a magic wand and turn me into a fairy princess—in a golden costume—*a poem she had written once. Only it had been part of a play. A coke dealer was going to produce it. The point was, she had eighteen of these prince charmings, each giving her a different colored costume; no wonder she was so god-damned confused. Each time one left she went back to being a black animal, no matter how each had dressed her. It had gotten to the point where she couldn't even relate to the tapping on the head, to the singing of the tune, to the presented flowers.

The ex-hippie remembered his acid trips and told her it could get worse, which she knew was true. The psychiatric social worker told her things could get better, but she knew they hadn't. She sat in a mental hospital and despaired: where could she go, what could she do, what kind of jobs could she get. When she came out with hope, feeling elated, she crashed; the last time she had left in despair, knowing there was no reason to get hopeful. Why build up again in order to fall.

Nowhere in the psychology books—she had read all of them—was it written "depressed people don't want to take care of themselves; they want other people to take care of them," but in her head she chastised herself for this constantly. Rarely was she aware of the shop windows she passed on the streets. Her voice churned with her advice to herself so that she never noticed the details, when she used to walk with such awe, experiencing the sensuality of the New York streets.

2

She sat with her mother's cleaning lady at the mahogany dining room table playing cards. "Charlena," she had said, "I see how people become alcoholics."

"What you need," Charlena had answered, "is to believe in Jesus and fall in love with a good man."

"Charlena," she had answered, "please, I can't stand it. I don't want to hear it. This is how I became schizophrenic. I can't take any more useless advice in. I'm so desperate I jump on all of it. So I tune out."

Tired of deliberating over decisions constantly, she had flipped a coin between being a bag lady (which would happen if she stayed in New York) and permanent institutionalization.

It was either men or mental hospitals, she had said to the psychiatric social worker before she left, and he had admired her capacity to be dramatic.

"But," she had protested "that is my sickness."

He had given her that irritated look, and left her when she said sex was a senseless activity, and besides, her roommates wouldn't allow it.

"If I want passion," he had said to her, "I have to go elsewhere apparently."

"What people don't understand," she had said listlessly, "is that my brilliance is hot flashes."

"That's what you get for trying to be a perfectionist." He had zipped up his pants, put on his black leather jacket, and left.

"See, even your friends get bored with you," her New York shrink had said. "And how are you going to go to social work school and help other people if you cry at yoga class. Besides, there are no jobs."

She had cried then, too: That's what she got for sitting in a mental hospital trying to "find a direction, rechannel her energies, figure things out. . . , exposing herself to stupid people who said "don't go, stay here 'til you learn to communicate with your parents." Twenty-year-old psych tech stuff. Like a chameleon, she got contaminated by the influence of all the various people.

And here she was.

Charlena had gone to buy her peanuts and cigarettes. She had typed the story. Activity therapy. Like handwashing, ritualistic activity. And what about a job. Maybe at the post office. Maybe she could make postcards. Maybe, maybe—but obsessional personalities cannot tolerate uncertainty and ambiguity.

"You see, Charlena, wherever I am, I am falling apart and I know I'm not right. And like it or not my parents have to take responsibility for me."

3

"Well," the psychiatrist had said. "It's been a while since I've seen you."

"I decided it didn't really matter where I was a mental patient." She had found out she would be one wherever she was.

"Yes it does. I won't abandon you. I'll be an anchor for you."

"All you have to offer is conversations. Maybe I'll go back to New York."

"Aren't you escaping?"

This was how she got to the point where she couldn't talk. Everything she said was put down from the outside.

"You are having trouble accepting that you are a mental patient."

Why shouldn't she?

4

Flashes of absurdity were in danger of popping out of her at all times. Here she was sitting in a bar in her home town with a security guard she had met while in the hospital.

He fashioned himself on the fact that they called him Crazy Pete on the local campus. He spoke a weird dialect of his own, infected with street slang from out east which he used, no doubt, trying to impress her. His fiancée had committed suicide driving a car, no longer being able to tolerate her life as an alcoholic. He was going to make a lot of money in computer sciences, or scuba diving, but music was his first passion. Bongo drumming. He didn't have much of a social life and was glad she was here for a year or two to settle down. He was tickled to have somebody around who didn't think him a gadabout as they thought of him at the university.

She thought him dumb, naive, obnoxious. Especially as he described his female drumming teacher "waving her tits and ass" at him as he played, sleeping with the head of the department at the university to get her position. Her feminist consciousness pricked at the story, immediately siding with the poor woman.

But blunt, blunt, blunt yourself constantly, she reminded herself, or else they'll put you in the hospital. This is what is known as adjusting to the limits of a small environment, what her father had said the hospital had tried to teach her.

At just that moment, he sensed she was thinking and interrupted her: "You and I, we think alike. We do the same kind of thinking."

"What?" she had said.

"Creative, avant garde, intellectual."

"No, mine is circular, disorganized, confused, not in touch with reality, not strategic or linear."

She ate the popcorn listlessly, allowed him to treat her to a video game, listening to him talk about how macho he was, thinking what a mess his cheap little dingy apartment near the hospital had been. "Why," she had said when she had seen it, "if you keep your room at the hospital like this they won't let you go to group two or group one, even though you don't have the slightest interest in either one."

He had hedged, laughed at her. She told him she felt like she was in a mental hospital no matter where she was, so demoralized had she become, and he was beginning to believe her.

She had gone to keep her appointment with the psychiatrist. She had refused to talk and merely dropped off a thirteen-page letter.

Crazy Pete had taken her for a ride in his red souped-up convertible when she came out.

▲ ▲ ▲

And this is what I get, she had thought, *for giving up my writing in the hopes of becoming middle class and respectable. I became labeled and became a lunatic in the process.*

Yet this Crazy Pete with the curly black locks and the blue bandanna scarf that made him look like a Hoosier roadman was the object of her current fantasies. Actually, no matter what the object, her fantasies were always similar. It didn't take much of an object to set them off. They would, in the words of the psychiatrist, "build a stable relationship." In her own image, this meant she would make love to him, her hands tied behind her back. She would read him her stories. He would come and rescue her from her parents' house. She would run away to his apartment when her brother and his wife and the kids came

down for the Seder, only coming back protected by Pete for the
dinner. She would move in with him. She didn't say all that, but
only, later, as he dropped her off, "Would you like me to clean
your apartment this weekend?" A joke in itself. Her mother had
made rules about how she was to change her sheets weekly,
empty the ashtrays of cigarettes, unpack her bags rather than
live out of suitcases, clean up the kitty litter, sweep, open the
windows, vacuum. Here she was, chastised as the family bum
derelict slob, offering to clean up this shrimp's apartment.
Sometimes—most of the time—she wondered, was it any
wonder, about herself.

▲ ▲ ▲

Ah ha! a shrink would say, if she bothered to tell the story
to anybody, *an inability to tolerate opposites! A borderline
symptom, a mark of personality disorganization. You must find
something between creativity and charwoman, between the
mountain climber and the traditional female. You have trouble
accepting that different parts of yourself coexist. Either/or, a
child's view of the world, you think in totalities or opposites.
Ah yes, you use childish defenses, you are primitive.*
     All they were was conversations, and she was sick of them.
     They had made her a cripple, unable to do, think, walk, talk,
so constricted was she by the labeling, the girdle.
     A captive in a captured land, chasing the myth of stability.
     It wasn't that she wasn't in touch with reality. She was very
much in touch with reality indeed, and she was sick of it.
     And the hospital had sickened her further.

5

     She began to drink all morning and lie around naked in the
sunroom of her mother's house watching movies on television
about husbands whose political careers had been ruined by
wives who became alcoholics. She had the need to communicate.
Yes, the lines kept zinging into her head, and the need for
achievement and the need for association. Trouble was, she
couldn't take a step, make a step, without wondering *Does this
get my human needs met* and she woke up screaming in the
middle of the night: "NO WONDER MY HUMAN NEEDS
CAN'T GET MET. I HAVE THE NEEDS OF A CHILD."

"But every one of us has a child inside," the psychiatrist would assure her, "and that's OK. You're the one who thinks it's not."

So she lay around the sunroom in her mother's house, wondering how she could tell Pete that she wasn't interested in sex, that she thought sex was a senseless activity. He thought they "thought alike" because she used the word "fuck" in her writing and when she got exasperated. But actually, she got repelled and changed the channels even when a sex scene came on the TV. She thought of being with the one who tried to save her with ideas about Jesus, and hearing his friend say, "You better get your diaphragm on sweetheart, he needs it." And that she was even in the situation was what made it more ridiculous.

Sex was ridiculous, but could she tell Pete? That would make him leave her. She needed somebody outside her mother's house to talk to, but as she had felt with the psychiatric social worker back in New York, must she prostitute herself for companionship (she had given up on the idea of comfort). No, that seemed crazy. Although maybe not. When she had been raped, she had had the same feeling of "prostituting herself on the mere glimmer of a hope that she would stay alive"; and she had felt shamed and guilty then too. When actually, maybe the use of sex was a survival instinct.

She knew she was lapsing into paralysis, unable to figure anything out, so she rolled over on her back to catch the rays of sun better and made herself get specific rather than vague and general in her memories. The danger of abstract thinking, she remembered, was something about which she had been very naive. Dissociated personalities turn to abstract thought and cling to it constantly. *Get specific, get specific, feel the sun on your body, let the TV in, and at least get specific in your reverie.*

She had run into the psychiatric social worker in the streets, in Brooklyn. She had been putting signs up trying to get typing work in the neighborhood. She had talked about applying for social work school, leaving out a few details such as being hospitalized four times and jumping the fence to get away, sick to death of being herded around like an animal and treated like a child and being told she couldn't make decisions for herself. He had offered to write her a letter of recommendation and to feed her. He had taken her back to his three-story brownstone where he lived with his wife and a baby daughter adopted from Colombia. He had fed her turkey and cranberry sauce (it was right after Thanksgiving) and remembered her romantically from when she had been active in political circles. "People always thought of you as scattered," he reassured her, "but affectionately, because as a writer you were so productive."

Within two hours, during which she had tried not to talk, he had diagnosed her as having a severe depression and said he wouldn't be surprised if she had made a few suicide attempts (four, she didn't say, including one the previous week) and recommended that she increase her social life. She had misunderstood that to mean he would invite her to dinners with his family and parties. She had felt comforted, and then she had refocused a bit in order to listen to him.

". . . preferably with someone safe, like a married man . . ."

"Are you volunteering yourself for the position?" she asked, out of scorn, shocked at him.

"Do you want to go upstairs?" Helplessness must be a turn-on to him, she mused, thinking how he looked like her grandfather. It's erotic, a woman in need—and his wife is so god-damn organized and efficient. She tried to refocus her thinking again to listen to him.

He went on mumbling about his recent theories, mobilizing specific anxiety rather than avoiding situations which created stress, increasing this, decreasing that, saying everything the exact opposite from the psychiatrist in the hospital who used to talk about building stable relationships, based not on sex, but on other "human bonds." The psychiatrist would talk loftily about life and what could be possible for her, needs for such and such, needs for this and this, the line they use in mental hospitals . . . and then she would come out of his safe little office onto the ward (euphemistically called "the unit") and the staff would be saying, "Do something physical, do something physical." "I don't feel like it." "You might enjoy it."

So, maybe she would, here. Sex was doing something physical, she reasoned. And besides she also heard the voice of the psychiatrist in her head. "You seem to be unable to get what you can from a situation. . . ."

"No," she finally answered the psychiatric social worker before her. "I don't have my diaphragm with me."

"Then let's go back to your place. Have an orgy with your roommates."

He evidently saw the gray look on her face turn grim.

"Just a fantasy. Not serious."

"Well," she deliberated. Do something physical, mental hospital advice number one; and number two, get what you can out of a situation. She had to go to Manhattan to put up more signs. She'd get him to walk her the seven blocks to her home, at least, her mind labored desperately, and she'd only have two more to the subway line then. Maybe she could do that alone, she consoled herself.

6

She deliberated over everything constantly because nothing did make sense, nothing did do any good, nothing ever turned out right that she initiated on her own. So she clung to the various people around her, and she continued to float. In New York it had been the string of them: the ex-hippy, the white-haired one, the one who believed in Jesus, the psychiatric social worker. Here it was to Crazy Pete and to her mother's cleaning lady. And at times to her mother and father. Either one of them would notice that she hadn't gone out of their house or been dressed for a few days and suggest that she accompany them somewhere—to run errands, to look at an apartment, to the bakery. They tried to ignore her habit of obsessively writing notes and cards to the psychiatrist. If she strained, she could find a pattern, a thread, some explanation, something, meaning. She was just trying to organize her mind, she would say to them. Her mother would look at her wearily. Her father would tilt his head, pat her on the back and say, "That's all right, you need a year to rest. Is there anything I can do for you sweetheart?"

▲ ▲ ▲

The sun shot across her back, and she felt good. She opened up her pink kimono bathrobe to feel it all the better. Might as well enjoy the present as well as she could.

And Pete, who had been calling her every night on the phone when he knew her parents were out of town, cut back to once a week when he knew they had come back from vacation (*bar mitzvahs* in Chicago in temples overlooking the lake, and then Louisville for her mother's professional psychology meetings: "Living with the Chronically Mentally Ill," the title of her mother's presented paper).

Was she supposed to trust him? Or could she not trust men because she couldn't trust her mother as a child? He had spoken on the phone about making $40,000 over the summer on a scuba diving job. The thought triggered the area that used to contain feeling in her head: *well, why get attached to this one, in a couple of months he'll be leaving me.* She had answered ruefully, *that's like guys on the in-patient unit, talking about getting a pickup truck and heading out west. The favorite fantasy of all of them. It's a dream.*

And she had hung up the phone before she had time to scream.

7

Then she had dinner with her father.

"Stop introducing me to everyone," she had said.

He looked at her strangely. He had introduced her to the waitress and to the people who worked in his office, as "my daughter."

"What did you do today?" he asked her.

Fell into a trance in the psychiatrist's office, she should have answered, talking about how everything was pointless, meaningless, how things spiralled around in her head and at least the writing helped to pin things down, except she had nobody to write to, no connecting conversations to other people in her head. Let alone connections to an audience.

Of course, she had been the one to break things off.

Instead, they had an argument about why she was like this.

"Like what?" The way she was.

"You mean sick?" he had asked her. "Probably because you can afford to."

Damn, here was a lecture coming. When if it was just money, she would be able to do something about it. Sure enough.

". . . You can do anything you want to do," when she tuned back in, he was scolding her.

"You think I want to be like this?"

"Like what?"

"A mental patient."

"I don't know what a mental patient is."

Here we go again, the verbal bantering, she thought, and tried to eat the steak in front of her. The problem with spending time with the members of her family was she could see where everything that was wrong with her had come from. The backs and forths; the overconsiderations; the questioning of her perceptions, decisions, and abilities; the communication that she was worthless, useless, scum; and an insincere veiled benign neglect for her.

She phoned an ex-mental-patient she had met on the ward, trying to seek safer connections. His mother had answered; Hank had been out of the house. "He sits in the living room. I say Hank, talk to me. He answers, 'Mother, I don't have anything to say.'" Yes, debilitated mental patients get like that. She had left her number. Hank had called her back. "Chasing any more rainbows lately?" Neither one had very much to say.

She went to sleep that night, tuning out the railings against her father, and dreamt about her book. The only published one.

8

Life was a carousel, only she had fallen off it. What was her fantasy now? That her mother's sunroom would disconnect from the house and float out to sea, lulled by the cooling of the dialogues of the ever-present movies on TV. Around the deck above the sunroom as it coasted out would be . . . psychiatrist after psychiatrist listening to her automatic hypno-reverie.

"BETTY BETTY GET UP GO UPSTAIRS. DO YOU WANT ME TO CARRY YOU?" Her father was yelling at her, wanting her to go upstairs. "THAT WAS ONE OF THE RULES. AREN'T YOU GOING TO FOLLOW IT?"

"I want to sleep by the TV. I like the continuous sounds that are always there to comfort me," she answered.

"I DON'T WANT YOU DOWN HERE."

"I want to be here. You don—"

9

"He wanted to carry you," mused the psychiatrist, carefully.

"Yes. I looked up in shock. I couldn't quite believe what he was saying to me."

"What did you say?"

"No. No, I said. OK, then I'll sit up and watch the TV, though why people can't lie around and sleep on couches is beyond me."

"Sounds pathological to me."

"It may be. He may be pathological, wanting to carry me. But I am the one who is in and out of mental institutions."

"It doesn't seem fair, does it?" the psychiatrist prodded her.

"That's what another of my shrinks has said. I have an immature sense of justice, apparently."

No. It wasn't fair. But who said life was fair. And what could she do about it. Write a letter to her New York shrink: *Dear Doris. I knew it was wrong to come out here. What about setting priorities. Contingency plans. Seeking sources of support both emotional and economic separate from my family. Mobilizing resources. My father is pathological. I am getting worse by being with him.*

Or to the psychiatric social worker, who, when last seen, had just put on his black leather jacket and zipped up his pants. *Yes, Jeffrey, I am descending deeper into the pathology as you predicted. I am drinking constantly and taking medication. Forgetting the vitamins you bought me. They are in my stuff somewhere. In storage. I haven't even unpacked. Baking, always. Eating muffins. Several varieties. Feeding chicken soup to my pathological parents. The shrink here is a subjectifying man; the one in New York, an objectifying woman. You were right. I needed something in the middle. Am getting worse, worse, worse.*

Or, merely touch up her novel, perfect the craft, develop the technique, make a story of it, to distance herself, build on her manuscript previously. Come to a synthesis. Make the connections.

But she could do any of the above, any of it, the writing in letters, prose, novels—when she thought communication worth it. Now she thought communication worthless. As was everything else apparently.

10

She resorted to the stationery store, and actually paid twelve of her last dollars to print up little stamps so she could get it out. DON'T TRUST SHRINKS, EVER AGAIN. I HATE MY MOTHER I HATE MY FATHER I HATE MYSELF. DON'T MAKE FRIENDS. AVOID THE INFLUENCE OF PEOPLE. DON'T SOLICIT REASSURANCES. BE PASSIVE. BE OBEDIENT. SHUT UP AND DO WHAT YOU'RE TOLD.

Thinking of money, she had tried to strike a deal with the printer. She would think up catchy slogans, like LOVE IS A TRAP, DON'T FALL INTO IT. He would print them. She would make 50% of all sales.

"You are not serious," he reassured her.

"Yes I am."

She had forgotten the seriousness of her sickness. She had lost all perspective. The idea had seemed relevant, worthwhile. It wasn't apparently.

11

"They've got me right where they want me, in a funny way," she said to the psychiatrist the next day.

"Oh, how is that?"

"I should get you books to read on the Jewish family. They never wanted me to get away. When I would come back from New York to visit, I'd try to get out of the house for a while—just to see high school friends—and my father would have to drive me there in the car, I'd have to go in, and get the girlfriend to come to their house to visit."

She paused, remembering some of the people she had met in the hospital. "I am no different than the fellow with the sunken cheeks who has been in the halfway house for ten years, who gets so flustered when his parents come to visit he sputters, or refuses to speak."

"We are all unique," the psychiatrist tried to suggest to her, but she didn't listen.

". . . or that Tim River, who lives out with his mom and dad in the small room right on the edge of Illinois. Was it Marshall? His mother never let him get away, and he is still living there. The only difference between me and the other mental patients is that I know better. Why, anybody who knows half of what I do stays away from the family."

"Maybe you can separate while you stay with them," he proffered hopefully, as he was wont to. Again she ignored him.

". . . yes," she continued her musing, "I hope they are happy. They've got what they always wanted, me trapped inside of their house. Not moving. No friends, no acquaintances, no contacts."

"Don't they want you to have your own life?"

"Not actually. Oh, am I going to sit here in Indiana and hate my parents, or try to get away. Is that called escape? I think it's healthy."

12

"I'm in my male drag state," she said to him, wanting to run up to him as he got off the bus and proclaim *Pim! Let's get*

*married! Stay here for a year and we'll work on our relationship!
You could go to graduate school at the university, while I do
what the doctor says, focus on the basics, earning a living. Here!
I bought us a gold ring, or rather I stole this brass ferrule from
the hardware store!* He hugged her and she concluded,
"Femininity is for fags." She was wearing her young, adolescent,
angry look, which she tried to hide behind her dark glasses, navy
sailor jacket, red beret, blue jeans, stompers. Didn't make a hit
with her mother or with anyone except men looking for loose
women around this Midwestern town.

He had just gotten off the bus from Cheyenne, Wyoming,
en route to New York from Frisco. Her old friend, the black gay
jazz musician. Also a poet. He had called her just after her
parents left town again, the previous night. Again the fantasies
of escape, rescue. Only Pim and she had known each other in
and out, over the years.

13

That too was fantasy. In reality he hadn't come. Calling her
from New York the next day, when he was supposed to be en
route to her from Chicago. "I don't want to be used as an
escape," he had said. She slammed down the phone, went to the
library to do research again.

Power, she decided, was the ability to turn your fantasies
into reality.

She called up Pete.

They joked. How would she make money. Offering
absurdity training courses at the university. She would bill
herself as a black surrealist writer of Jewish heritage in a Bible
Belt town. She would train the frat boys in categories of lines to
use at parties, each of which had come to her in what she
referred to as her absurdity flashes which, when they first
started, she had hoped would be a play.

Number 42: Listen to 'em talk.

Number 35: Find her fantasy and feed it.

Number 97: Perhaps I could be of some assistance.

He laughed, letting her know he appreciated her.

They met for a drink.

She moved in with him.

PSYCHIATRY NITTY GRITTY

Clover

Sheltered by no port
Far from a shoreline
A naiveté
Is dropped overboard

Keelhauled down
Shrunk and scourged
Through barnacles
And murk of algae
Zag zig zag zag
In mindrake
Water of lies
To surface bailing
Alone in a sieve
Grasping a lifeline
Of fanged seaweed

Occasionally
A bird flying over
Plops a message

PART 2

BUT IT DOESN'T HAVE TO BE FOREVER

The controversy surrounding the efficacy of psychiatric medicine has been going on for more than three decades. Psychiatrists themselves admit that they don't know what "mental illness" is; nevertheless, their opinions continue to be sought, their theories practiced, their methods employed. Moreover, psychiatric treatment can be forced upon individuals without due process of law even though, as activist Ellen Field points out, "There is no evidence to show that they [the psychiatrists] have any indisputable knowledge at all."*

There is, in fact, a growing body of evidence bringing the value of psychiatric medicine into question.** Furthermore, more often than not, this "medicine" is a complete atrocity—comparable only to the history out of which it grew: Is four-point restraint—being tied down at the wrists and ankles—an improvement over being bound with chains? Is the cage inhumane whereas the seclusion room is not? Are the deaths that result from the use of neuroleptic drugs better than the deaths that resulted from bloodletting? Is the terror inspired by the passing of electric current through the brain an improvement over the shock of being submersed in ice water? Are the side effects of today's treatments (it would take pages to

---

* Ellen Field, *The White Sheets* (Los Angeles: Tasmania Press, 1964).
** See Peter Breggin M.D., *Toxic Psychiatry* (New York: St. Martin's Press, 1991).

list them all) better? Is the brain damage caused by psychiatric "medicine" better now?

For many of us who have been personally subjected to these practices, the realization of society's wholesale acceptance and/or ignorance of them is intolerable. The torture of those who have been labeled "mentally ill" is not a thing of the past: it is happening *now*. The methods have changed over the years, but the cruelty is the same.

For those who may be tempted to argue that such treatment is justified by the threat of violence by "mental patients," the fact is that those labeled "mentally ill" are not a particularly violent group of people: in the words of Ellen Field, "We are sheep, not rebels."* Nevertheless, the debilitating effects of some mental and emotional distresses and the extreme suffering often associated with these might lead some to wonder: If not the current mental health system, what then?

There are many survivors of psychiatric treatment who have found alternatives to the current mental health system. We have done what many in psychiatry would say is impossible: We have taken the mystery out of "madness," defined it in our own terms, and made our lives to suit our own purposes. And despite gloomy psychiatric prognoses, we have come out with flying colors, empowered and whole.

Out of our shared respect for personal eccentricity and nonconformity have come a variety of alternatives: From survivor-run drop-in centers to peer support groups to alternative medicine. Like the shamans of tribal cultures, many of us have found that the best healers are the "wounded" healers, those who have "been there" and gotten through it. And the best healing is that which comes from respecting mental, emotional, physical and spiritual processes, and in the light of that respect, *exercising our right to choose what works best for each of us as individuals*.

The following pages contain the testimonies of women who've taken control of their own lives.

---

* Ellen Field, *The White Sheets* (Los Angeles: Tasmania Press, 1964).

RESPECTING OUR DIFFERENCES

Jeanine Grobe

During the process of compiling this section of the anthology, I sent a questionnaire to the writers requesting information about the alternatives they were using. The results were surprising because there was little consensus of experience among us.*

Some women reported that self-help groups were helpful to them; others felt they weren't. The same was true for peer support/co-counselling, drop-in centers, spiritual practices, political activism, creative/artistic pursuits and new belief systems. Where alternative medicine was concerned, the reports showed that many of us were using these approaches, to one extent or another, but we're using different ones for different purposes. Some of these included herbalism, Shamanism, homeopathy, nutrition, relaxation and visualization techniques, bodywork, dancing, martial arts, meditation, walking, exercising and spending time in nature. Once again, there were conflicting reports. Some women, for example, found meditation was helpful while others found it wasn't.

Our ways of dealing with depression, anxiety, confusion, fear, sadness/grief, "hallucinations," and so on, reflected highly personal preferences ranging from wearing particular articles of

---

* The author wishes to acknowledge the following women for participating in the questionnaire: Kris Yates, Clover, Batya Weinbaum, Beth Greenspan, Barbara Peller, and Sylvia Caras.

clothing, to setting boundaries with family members, to staying out of public places.

The picture that emerged from the results of this questionnaire, and from the conversations I've had with many of us over the years, is that the process of healing is as individual as we ourselves are. Maybe the only "medicine" we can all be sure to benefit from is the respect for who we are as individuals. While some of us have some things in common, we are not all in the same place at the same time.

▲ ▲ ▲

In my own experience, healing was a very personal thing that involved coming to trust myself. I wish I could say that it involved the complicated, theoretical know-how of some brainy physician; that would be, if not simple, at least expected. The truth is that my healer came from the opposite end of the spectrum. She was a shaman, which, by psychiatric standards, would be considered "mentally ill."

When I met this woman, I was a mess. A constant, excruciating anxiety over the course of several months had caused me to lose over twenty-five pounds. The outer world was a painful nightmare of sounds, shapes, and stimuli that tortured every nerve in my body; my senses were so acute that everything took on a cartoon-like character of diabolic proportions. My emotional state vacillated between terror and apathy, which, on occasion, was relieved by anguish and desperation.

The first time I met this woman, I bombarded her with my fears and concerns. About halfway through, she interrupted me saying, "Do you mind if we go outside? I'm sensitive to what you're feeling and I'm a little dizzy."

This was a new experience for me. Never had a "professional" person been *that* sensitive to me, let alone *honest* about her own vulnerability. We went outside and sat on the ground under the trees while I continued.

Several times she interrupted me again to say, "I understand about that." This was different too. She wanted me to know that she understood about some things—as if she knew no one else ever had, as if she knew how much I needed to hear that. And the most puzzling thing was that she meant it.

Before I left, she said, "You're suffering so much, you need something to help you feel good. Would you like a book to read?" A book? No one had ever prescribed a book before. "This one is pretty good," she said as she handed me a book I would not soon forget, *The Daughters of Copperwoman* by Anne Cameron.

I read the book over the next few days and it was the first light-flicker I'd seen in months. I was reading about Native American women in unbearable, impossible circumstances, and I could relate to them. I had read hundreds of books before that one; philosophy had been my favorite subject; it appealed to my thinking. But this was different. This book made me *feel* good. I could relate to what the women in it were going through and I felt connected to them. What was more, I felt understood.

The woman who gave me this book, as I said, was a shaman. I could tell you what that means in dictionary terms, but it would be truer to tell you what it meant from my experience.

It meant that unlike the psychiatrists who had treated me for seventeen years:

▲ She did not equate my "symptoms" with "mental illness." (I learned to see myself as not sick.)

▲ She had experienced these "symptoms" herself and had no fear of them. (I learned to relate to my own experiences without fear.)

▲ She related to me not from textbook knowledge nor from "clinical experience," but from her *own* experience, thus enabling her to be spontaneous. (I learned to trust her.)

▲ She valued my integrity over anything else, and never presumed to know what was "best for me," let alone force me into something against my will, which would have been the complete antithesis of what she stood for. (I learned to trust myself.)

▲ Through my own experiences, she showed me how to fashion tools with which to take care of myself. (I became powerful.)

▲ Sometimes she asked *me* to help *her*, not because she was using psychology to get me to feel better about myself, but because she *honestly* wanted my help. (I learned my own value.)

▲ She was not afraid of me so she accepted *all* of me. (I learned to accept myself.)

This woman helped me realize that regardless of how "abnormal" or "unusual" or "out of the ordinary" my experiences were, according to someone else's ideas, I was okay. That made the difference for me. Today I've accepted my "wrong" feelings, my "crazy" experiences and "bizarre" thinking and everything else I was told was not "right" about me. And while my choices have become more specific, I have become present in all of them.

If there is anything I have learned, it is that we need to be true to ourselves. And this is true for everyone, not just survivors of the mental health system. But it's not always easy to do. The pressure to conform to one thing or another hits us at every turn. If you have the added burden of being plagued with self doubt, that pressure can set you at odds with yourself without your even realizing it. That is why it is so important to respect our differences.

We each have the right to form our own opinions regardless of what anyone else tells us. And we need not account to anyone for our beliefs.

Survivor activist John Stuart has written a wonderful set of rights that has helped me many times. I'd like to end by quoting a portion of it, which affirms the mental freedoms that are our birthrights:[*]

▲ The right to have and hold my own ideas and opinions about anything.

▲ The right to talk about my ideas and opinions.

▲ The right to keep to myself my ideas and opinions.

▲ The right to think about and form and choose my ideas and opinions in my own way and in my own time.

▲ The right to keep to myself my reasons for my choice of ideas and opinions.

▲ The right to change my ideas and opinions.

▲ The right to agree with and accept other people's ideas and opinions.

▲ The right to disagree with and reject other people's ideas and opinions.

▲ The right to make sense of my life in my own way, in my own words, for my own purposes.

---

[*] John Stuart's complete list of rights (numbering more than thirty and growing) can be obtained in his 'zine by writing to Madhouse Exit, P.O. Box 7652, Santa Cruz, CA 95061. Rights reprinted here by permission of John Stuart.

As survivors of the mental health system, we have choices. There were times when it was hard for me to realize that, but it is now part of my own personal medicine. The place to start is where you are.

BEARING WITNESS

Why the Personal Can't Help Being Political[*]

Janet Gotkin

This title isn't quite accurate. The personal isn't always political. It doesn't *become* political UNTIL YOU TELL SOMEONE. If you keep your story locked away, if you never share it, never take the risk of exposing it to the light of day, it eats away at you in your isolation and aloneness. It yields little more than turmoil, conflict, anger, and grief. The memories turn on themselves, wrapping sorrow into intricate balls of pain. There is suffering, regret, self-blame, and rage. Pain and more pain. Rarely is there liberation. Never is there empowerment. Your story remains just that—YOUR STORY—yours and yours alone.

When you take that awesome, scary jump and TELL YOUR STORY, then, then—all sorts of miraculous things happen. And the first is the transformation of the personal to the political. No, you don't automatically decide to run for office. Not that kind of political. Political in its purest sense.

Political comes from the Latin word *politicus* meaning "the people." When you share your story, whatever it may be, that act of courage and generosity allows you to transcend your own pain. The gift of your story—and that is what it is, a

---

[*] Keynote speech presented at the annual Meeting of the National Association of Rights, Protection, and Advocacy (NARPA), Kansas City, MO, November 13, 1992.

gift—becomes an infusion of strength and clarity for others. It is a gift to a community of sufferers and strivers for change. It is another thread in the growing communal quilt of survivor stories, and ultimately your thread adds color and life and strength to that quilt and forges an unbreakable bond with other survivors. Your story, when you tell it, ends your isolation forever; it joins you with others. It—the act of telling—makes you political. And you will never be as alone as you were before you told.

That is what happened to me when I wrote *Too Much Anger, Too Many Tears.* But it was my early and tentative experiences in the mental patients' movement, in 1971 and 1972, that prepared me to become political and helped me to get ready for the act of self-revelation that was *Too Much Anger, Too Many Tears*.

In the fall of 1970, I nearly died from a huge overdose of Mellaril. I was in a coma for five days, and I emerged, amazingly, and found myself drug free, for the first time in almost ten years. I had a flash of vision in the days following my emergence from the coma, and I KNEW—I don't know how I knew—that if I didn't get away from New York, from my parents, and, most of all, from my psychiatrist, I would end up in a hospital again and I would die, from the drugs and shock or, eventually, from a successful suicide attempt.

Paul and I sold all of our belongings, took our kitten Jenny with us, and went to live in Paris for as long as our money would hold out. During the ten months we spent in France, I did a lot of thinking, a lot of feeling, and a lot of reading—R.D. Laing, Erving Goffman, Thomas Szasz. I was trying to understand what had happened to me—how I could have been a hard core "mental patient" for almost ten years, in and out of hospitals, recipient of every known psychoactive drug that existed at the time, in huge doses and combinations, subject to more than 100 electroshocks, a "mental patient" everyone was describing as hopeless—and then, one day, after a massive drug overdose and a nearly deadly coma, emerge as "normal" or "cured." It was

---

* Janet Gotkin and Paul Gotkin, *Too Much Anger, Too Many Tears: A Personal Triumph Over Psychiatry*, reprinted by New York: Harper Perennial, 1992.

strange and perplexing. I didn't understand and I wanted to understand. I felt that my life depended on my understanding.

When we came back to the United States in the late summer of 1971, a friend told me about a group that was meeting in New York City called Mental Patients Resistance.* My friend gave me a telephone number and I called, my heart beating so hard I thought I would die on the spot. The person I spoke with, who would truly change my life, was Judi Chamberlin. I don't remember what I told her; I have no idea what she said to me. But I do know that later that week I drove from Croton, where Paul and I had just moved, to an apartment in Brooklyn Heights, and attended my first meeting of ex-patients, a "consciousness-raising" session.

I listened really hard that night. I don't think I said very much. But I came away with the absolutely clear and unshakable belief that my life was about to take a radical turn—and that if I followed the path that seemed to be opening up for me, I would forever be a changed person. I wasn't sure who that new person would be. I wasn't even sure I was going to like the new person. I just knew that this path beckoned me with hope and promise. I wanted—I needed—to follow it.

A few weeks—maybe a month or so—later, I went to my first public meeting, after Judi assured me that if I sat on the stage, as part of the panel who were talking about their experiences in mental hospitals, I didn't really have to talk if I didn't want to. The meeting was in a basement (it seems to me, as I look back, that we went to a lot of meetings in basements) and was a discussion held after a Sunday service in some very liberal church that prided itself on nurturing liberation movements. In fact, the congregation of this very liberal church turned out to have an inordinate number of members of the so-called mental health professions, many of them psychiatrists, and they were not at all happy with what they heard that day.

Well, as you might guess, I did speak that afternoon. Haltingly, with great fear, I told my story publicly, for the very first time, and with my new knowledge that what had happened to me was not an isolated incident caused by my badness or

---

* By the way, for those of you whose historical memory doesn't extend to the early 1970s, there were *three* ex-inmate groups in New York City at that time—the heady early years of this movement!

sickness. I think I spoke fairly well, even as I waited for the sky
to fall or for the proverbial men in the white coats to come and
cart me away. (After all, I was publicly challenging the men who
had exercised so much power over me for so many years!) I even
engaged in a one-on-one argument with a psychiatrist who
challenged my assertion that electroshock was dangerous and
cruel. I stood my ground; I didn't let him badger me. I didn't
submit.

I don't know if I can really describe how I felt after that day.
Exuberant. Lightheaded. Triumphant. Strong. Free. Connected.
Perhaps most profoundly I felt connected to the people who
spoke with me on the panel and, in a broader sense, to the people
who were suffering indignities at the hands of psychiatry and
those who were trying to reclaim their lives.

For ten years I had felt shamed and isolated, fearful for my
sanity, humiliated that my behavior had caused the
well-meaning psychiatrists, in their efforts to "help me," to visit
such tortures upon me as Thorazine, Mellaril, Prolixin, and
electroshock, seemingly endless rounds of electroshock. When I
went to that first meeting in the small Brooklyn apartment, I
knew that, finally, I wasn't alone anymore. When I spoke out
and told my story, however briefly, I knew, without really
analyzing it, that I had done something more than just help
myself. I had offered my truth, my essence. Other people would
hear, would make connections, would not feel as scared and
isolated as they had. And maybe, maybe, they, too, would begin
to make sense of their experiences, and find power in their own
truths. Maybe, maybe, we could join our personal stories into
a powerful chain; from our collective truths we would bring
about change. It was a heady, scary, revolutionary prospect.

It was the impulse to share that lay behind my decision and
Paul's to tell our story. I knew that what I had learned from
listening to others—that I was not unique in my struggle to
survive the assaults of psychiatry—was important. We both felt
that the good that could come out of telling my story—actually
both of our stories—would far outweigh the privacy we would
forego if our book was published.

And, indeed, I feel that that has been the case. And it's not
because we're such good writers or because my story or Paul's
story is so unusual or so dramatic. It is, I believe, because there
is nothing more profoundly powerful than personal truth. In
fact, I believe that the power of personal narrative is so

monumental that over the years enormous efforts have been launched to minimize or undermine the veracity of people who would dare to tell their truth.

What can be so dangerous about one person's story—that causes whole institutions to muster massive efforts to discredit the teller? Why not ignore the teller? After all how can *one single person* influence *anything*?

I believe there is something almost mystical, almost magical in the potency of personal truth. I know, from the letters Paul and I have received over many years, what our truth has meant to so many people. My story, in *Too Much Anger, Too Many Tears*, has brought people into the light of awareness of the true nature and intent of the so-called mental health system. My story has mobilized people to action, has brought relief to people who thought they were all alone in their unique suffering, validation to people who believed they were, indeed, crazy, the way they had been told by psychiatrists. My story, which was once a closely held tale of personal torment, became a ray of clear light for many people, a document that engendered change, that gave courage and insight and renewed hope. *Our* story, *our* testimony, moved from being our private personal property to being the asset of a community, a resource for an entire movement. And the power of one became multiplied many times over: the personal truly became political.

That is the unique and awesome power of personal truth—that my story, your story, our stories—move other people to tell their stories—and after a while there is no way to avoid the massive truths of these accounts of people courageous enough to bear witness.

I was not easily believed or taken seriously when *Too Much Anger, Too Many Tears* was first published in 1975. For one thing, our book, which was hailed by *The New York Times Book Review* as "one of the most important documents in the history of psychiatry," was not reviewed in a single national publication outside the library field. No major book club would take us on (one asked us to change the ending in order to be included in their list), and there was no mass market paperback sale. Most network talk shows were reluctant to have us on to speak.

Representatives of the institutions under siege, institutional psychiatry, launched considerable efforts to discredit me, to undermine the power of this simple story. The tactics weren't subtle; you're all so familiar with them, you could probably say them as fluently as I can. In reviews in "professional" publications and in public appearances, the people who felt themselves under attack called me every name you could think of—implying that I made up most of what I wrote about, that I was so mentally ill I couldn't understand what had happened to me, that I was in denial about my mental illness and therefore didn't appreciate all the treatments I received, that my reports about the horror of drugs and ECT were, again, the product of my mental illness, that, in fact, I should attribute my "health" to the fine therapeutic efforts of the doctors. And on and on and on.

I've thought a lot about this process of attempted character assassination—where it comes from, what motivates it. I think the answer is really very simple. Elizabeth Packard expressed it most succinctly. Elizabeth Packard was an extraordinary nineteenth-century woman who was railroaded into a state mental asylum by her Calvinist minister husband, acting in collusion with the asylum superintendent. When she attempted to get her story out, started organizing the inmates, and protested her incarceration, the superintendent brought all his considerable power to bear, condemning her to the vilest, dirtiest, coldest portion of the basement of the institution, in the company of the most disturbed and neglected inmates. Writing of her experiences in a two-volume document called *Modern Persecution, Or Insane Asylums Unveiled*, Elizabeth Packard tells how she responded to a question from one of the nurses, as to why the head of the asylum was persecuting her so. She answered: "He perceives that I am a truth-telling woman, and he is afraid."

That, after all, is the heart of the matter: truth is powerful. Truth is so powerful that those who are threatened by even one single person's truth will take drastic measures to undermine its effects. Think about Anita Hill, and the wild efforts that were made to discredit her. She was called frustrated, crazy, scorned, sexually deviant, radical, irrational, vindictive, unstable—anything and everything—to cancel out the power of her truth. Clarence Thomas did get his Supreme Court appointment, but that was just politics—not the kind we're talking about here today. And for the first time in U.S. history, women found the courage, from listening to Anita Hill, to tell the truth about the pervasiveness of sexual harassment.

Lawmakers and employers and people in all segments of U.S. society were forced to begin to confront this long-suppressed issue—and all because one courageous woman told her truth.

Think about Sigmund Freud and his suppression of the seduction theory. Thanks to Jeffrey Masson's bold research and unswerving commitment to telling the truth, we know that in the early days of Freud's practice, he heard many stories from patients about how they had been sexually abused as children. He believed them. Why not believe them? But then Freud changed his story. He decided he didn't believe them. This widespread abuse didn't really happen, he decided; these people *fantasized* their abuse. If, in fact, the kind of abuse Freud was discovering was truly taking place, what did that mean for the sanctity of the family? What did it say about fathers? What kind of lies and distortions were holding up the very fabric of society? The reality of the pervasiveness of child sexual abuse was too revolutionary to be allowed to surface, so Freud chose to disqualify the witnesses by asserting that they were, in essence, making up their stories.

Jeff Masson's book *The Assault on Truth*[*] tells the sad, sordid tale of Freud's refusal to accept the truth of his patients' lives and outlines the far-reaching ramifications of this denial. The most horrific result of Freud's action was that until the early or mid-1980s almost no practitioner of psychotherapy believed any person who confessed to having been sexually molested as a child. Childhood sexual abuse just didn't exist.

And then, quite recently, something extraordinary happened. Adults, most but not all of them women, began remembering long-buried incidents of sexual abuse from their childhoods. And, most wonderful and startling of all, they began talking about it. They began telling their stories. And the telling of these stories by some gave others courage to share their personal tales, to come forward with the gifts of the pain from their lives. In unprecedented numbers, survivors of childhood sexual abuse are speaking truth to power and telling each other—and those of us who will listen—what happened to them when they were children.

---

[*] Jeff Masson, *The Assault on Truth: Freud's Suppression of the Seduction Theory* (New York: HarperCollins, 1992).

I have a particular interest in this avalanche of personal stories because two and a half years ago, I, too, began to regain some fragments of memories from my childhood, which had previously been shrouded in almost total darkness. Like thousands and thousands of adults now coming into possession of their childhood memories, I found out and now know that I am a survivor of years of repeated sexual abuse and brutal physical assault by my father and my older brother. I guess you might say I've experienced a real double whammy—I am a survivor of both incest *and* psychiatry. But I know that I am far from alone.

I must be very strong. We're all strong—us survivors. And it is our strength, as well as our determination to tell the truth, that scares the perpetrators and scares the keepers of the status quo. It is the power of our truth to empower others that scares them the most. And it should.

So, as it appears that both physical and sexual child abuse are a scourge in our society of unimaginable proportions, a new theory has emerged as a weapon in the battle to promote disbelief. It is called "false memory syndrome," and this is how it goes: people who say they remember being sexually abused as children are not to be believed because they are suffering from "false memory syndrome." (Even the efforts to discredit us bear a medical/psychiatric tinge these days!) According to this theory, the things people think they remember never happened but have been planted in their minds by therapists. Other variations of this theme accuse newly aware adults who accuse their perpetrators of being sick, crazy, vindictive, out of control. And journalists have become fond of calling the regaining of memories of childhood sexual abuse a "fad." Anything not to have to believe the survivors, not to have to face their truth.

It isn't really surprising. In fact, as I think about this, I find a kind of cosmic relief in realizing that the politics of power hasn't changed over the centuries. Even in ancient Greece, they were killing the messengers who brought bad news rather than facing the truth of their reports. On the one hand, incest survivors; eyewitness reporters of wartime atrocities; whistle-blowers like Karen Silkwood; involuntary inmates like Elizabeth Packard; ex-inmate activists who tell about the horrors of psychoactive drugs, the dangers of ECT, the crassness and venal misuse of power by psychiatrists—all have consistently received much the same fate—to be disbelieved and discredited, often by the most outlandish excuses—discredited because, like Elizabeth Packard, they—we—are too dangerous. On the other hand, all—even those who never intended to—have become agents of change, drawn along by the forces they've unleashed.

Anita Hill, who spoke out with great reluctance and then only to clear the record about Clarence Thomas—never intended to become the spokesperson for a movement. She clearly expected to give her testimony and return to her structured and predictable academic life in Oklahoma. But that isn't what happened. Anita Hill's story, like so many other survivors' stories, took on a political life of its own. As powerful as her individual testimony was, its impact was compounded a thousand times by the myriad stories of women who were moved by her honesty and courage, and who decided to risk derision and disbelief to speak out about their own experiences.

Anita Hill, the quiet, politically conservative law professor who never made waves over any issue and who supported the Republican agenda all of her adult life, now criss-crosses the nation, facilitating change, addressing the issue of sexual harassment with fervor and passion. Anita Hill—the reluctant organizer, the quintessential example of the personal become political. It doesn't even matter if she wanted or intended it to happen. It happened.

In much the same way, I have found myself, over the years, the unwilling focal point for communal desires for change. Yes, I wanted to tell my story. Yes, I thought it would be important. Yes, I felt I had a responsibility to be a witness—because I knew that I could be a compelling voice for the thousands of people who hadn't survived psychiatry—or who couldn't tell their own stories. But there have been times when I would have liked to have the luxury of a truly private life. There were times, when I was feeling tired and overwhelmed, I would have liked to see the process reverse itself—and the political become personal again. That just doesn't happen.

Our simple stories, our personal truths—each individual telling of pain or injustice—bears within it, once it is told—the power to alter history. Look what the truths told by psychiatric survivors have done in only twenty years—spawned a strong movement of community activists, created a system of protection and advocacy, created a literature of survivors, influenced legislation, and raised consciousness about the true nature of institutional psychiatry.

That is just the beginning. Much remains to be done, and I believe that the impetus behind the radical changes we envision—in the way we look at each other, the way we care for each other, and the way we divide power in our society—will come from the truths of people's lives, as they already have. Individual people speaking out, sharing, telling their stories. Emboldening and empowering other people. It can be—it will be—it *must* be—a firestorm of stories so unequivocally and irrefutably true and powerful that not all the efforts of all the psychiatric bureaucrats in all the hospitals and all the government departments and all the mental health clinics and research centers will be able to stop it.

It can—and does—start with a single experience, a single person's decision to break the silence and share a personal tale. The story of one person—like Elizabeth Packard or Anita Hill—becomes a communal treasure and moves other people to take the step of speaking out and becoming witnesses to their own pain. Each takes courage from the other, and soon we have broken the barriers that have prevented us from taking our power and realizing our collective strength.

As I drove to work yesterday, I was listening to an old Joan Baez tape, unregenerate folk music enthusiast that I am. She was singing one of my very favorite classic ballads, about a union man who was killed by the bosses and who went on to live in the hearts and wills and imaginations of succeeding generations that struggle to have their voices heard and their rights observed. As I listened to the story of Joe Hill, I found myself crying, because I *felt* his pain. I've known and sung about Joe Hill since I was a teenager, and I realized that I've carried the inspiration of Joe Hill with me for all those years. That is the power of one life to change many.

I believe that in all the struggles we are witness to and part of, to change the priorities of our society, to humanize our social system, to bring about nurturing and healing environments—in all of our struggles to gain recognition of our pain, validation of our experiences, justice for survivors—in all these efforts to defend our lives and ORGANIZE for change, we find that we have incorporated into our very being the contemporary Joe Hills—not necessarily martyrs, but witnesses—courageous, unyielding, undaunted by efforts to blot out their truths. Before there was legislation, before there was litigation, before government entered the picture to promote advocacy, before the foundation grants appeared and the community groups got started—before all the progress and change, there were the people who lived their pain and shared their stories.

Speaking out and sharing pain and oppression, simple acts of sharing, allowed me to transform my own personal pain into a vehicle for political empowerment and change. And not, as I said, because my story is unusually dramatic, rather because it's so common that it speaks to people whose pain has been private and silent and encourages them to give voice to their unique experiences, to share their lives. From those shared lives comes the truly unstoppable power to politicize, to organize, and, ultimately, to change the world.

HEALING AS A WAY OF LIFE

Myra Lilliana Splitrock

No, they never put rats in my vagina like they did to Chilean womyn during dictatorship. No, they never raped me, then tore open my womb, heavy with child like they did to the El Salvadoran womyn. No, they didn't round me up in a concentration camp, put a permanent number tattoo on my arm and gas all my family members like they did to Jewish womyn in Germany. No, I am not pregnant with my twelfth baby because my husband wants that. Neither have circumstances forced me into prostitution. I didn't have the bad luck to be born and grow up around drugs, extreme police brutality, or malnutrition as a kid. Neither did I suffer from racism except for the sadness I feel for the pain inflicted on womyn I love and admire, and the frustration I feel over the fact that it keeps us from working together easily to create a world that loves and respects all womyn, children, people and planet earth.

Lucky me, growing up in a white, catholic, respected, farmer's family in a small European village . . .

How nice to wrap up
all those sleepless nights
in one white academic word:
"dysfunctional family."
May she rest in peace.

Of course, it's not that simple. Neither is it a joke. More in than out of therapy the past twenty years, I have demystified my privileged life. Feminist activism has kept me more or less sane. Although I was born the year after World War II, and my country was at peace, my survival has been a war.

One incest survivor said, "Incest is like being run over by a gigantic truck, only no one notices it. The injuries are invisible."

A friend of mine, a psychology student, once suggested we do an association exercise about my father to discover why I acted strange around men—not falling in love with them. In the exercise, I associated my father with murder. The moment my friend asked if I wanted him to say the word, I got very scared but nodded my head. He said, "murderer." Something inside of me snapped, made a connection. I screamed "yes" and cried.

For days afterward, when I'd look into the mirror my eyes looked so sad. I felt such inside cold. All I could remember was being a little girl who couldn't even talk, could barely walk, when something had happened to me that had scattered me. . .

> in the mirror float
> blue pools still
> of loneliness and terror
> of a little girl that
> could hardly walk, talk
> age 1-1/2 she scattered
> into black
> stopped existing.

Incest and psychological child abuse have been denied and kept a shameful secret until recently. We need not be ashamed for the harm done to us as little girls. It was never our fault. Neither is it our fault that the world is so lesbophobic. It is no wonder that many survivors of incest became survivors of psychiatric oppression when so many parts of our reality were denied, had no words, didn't seem to exist; so one's problems seemed to be character defects and personal, as if male dominance and heterosexism aren't social diseases.

Woman-incest survivor-lesbian artist-warrior-writer-patriarchy-denial-sexism-lesbophobia-manipulation-indoctrination-classism-consumerism-racism-struggle-justice-human rights-transforming society-support groups-feminism. These are some of the concepts that give me understanding and strength, but I did not find them in the mental health system.

Psychiatric hospitals are emotional torture, nightmareland, hell. In concentration camps, one knows who the enemy is. In mental hospitals, the enemy is cloaked in condescending friendliness to help "poor you" who failed in the world; teach you "better ways to function"—to adapt to an authoritarian, sexist, racist, classist society.

Working class women of color are treated even worse, because to be admitted to a psychotherapeutic community you have to be able to talk their lingo. Mental institutions and Freudian therapy are institutions of control that damage and blame women, maintain patriarchal power structures. But feminists have developed alternatives because Goddess knows how many of us have been badly hurt from birth on. And it may well be the most sensitive and intelligent among us who dared resist and got burned most.

For me, it is involvement in the struggle for social change that gives me hope and strength. I need a world that appreciates all women and diversity. Each human being deserves respect and love, validation.

In learning to love myself, it helps if others do so too. I need a support group that understands me and I them. I need community, rituals, art. These nurture me, make me feel good about myself. I think that anything that makes you feel good about who you are, makes you feel proud of yourself, is healing.

I hurt for all my sisters in mental hospitals who were not so lucky to escape the net that robs souls and spirits, sucks them empty. After more than twenty years of never returning to the mental hospital, that world still scares me. I only spent 4 of my 46 years there, but many years struggling to never return.

At home, I make my altar for all compañeras who died. I put some photos on it and images of strong women, creative women. I put flowers and foods and favorite rocks, shells. I remember the many women who are war victims. Those for whom the pain of oppression was too much. I recommit myself today, again, to participate in the resistance and the global struggle of women to create a respectful, accepting, loving world who sees how precious each one is.

FOR CHILDREN
WHO KEEP BANGING

Bluebird

She is seventeen
  and bangs her head
on walls.
  She bangs her head
her hands until
  when they're
raw they tie her down.
They tie her down
  until when they can
do nothing with
  her they seclude her
in institutions
  where still nobody
can do nothing.
  They sign papers
tucking her
  down on table
leather straps
  and tie her brain
to the sound
  of a second
waves going
  through her head
they call electroshock.

  Each time
a little more
  electrocution

they carry her
  on carts
her heart
is damaged
  until there
is nothing
  more she
still bangs
  her head
until
  there is no more
thought
left
  is the way they
want her
  with no more
courage
  she has nothing
left
  her heart
is broken
  against the side
of her head.

It is like
the little
  girl
they left in
  a closet
and didn't
feed her
  and left
with not enough
she too
  a little
day each more
  she died
until she no
  longer
cried.

I watched

her then
just a little
girl, age twelve,
   and no more
nothing they could
   no more
   if they tried
do something more.
She died then
   a little girl
   not to cry
anymore,
   and like
I know these
   little girls
like I know
   myself
just crying
   and trying
to remember
   the last time
the leather
   strap came
down is when
   I started
banging back
   only my
head kept dying
is when the
   thought of
   death when
the hands reach
   out
only they're
so scarred
   from banging.

These little
   girls
keep calling me
   now.
Sometimes I wish

they'd stop.
Don't call me
Don't call me
but still the
   telephone rings
with a little
girl.
Somehow we together
   if we try
can call back
   to her.
Somehow if we
   stop sitting
here we can
   take away
the leather straps,
the metal plates,
   take away
the tables
and the empty
rooms and maybe
   together if we
   take away
all the
   empty answers
   and all the
filled up institutions
   maybe if we
keep trying to
   tear down
what people
don't know
   we can
reach out
   with our hands
if we get
   close enough to
Touch
   If we Touch
this is what we
   have
for children

who keep
banging.
This is the
   answer.

A DOUBLE WHAMMY

Sexism, Mentalism,*
and What We Can Do About It

Janet Foner

The women's movement has brought home to us the idea that the personal is political. This has certainly been true of my life as a "mental patient" and ex-"patient," or psychiatric survivor, as I prefer to call myself.

When I was twenty-one years old, in the year 1967, a series of circumstances led to my being "hospitalized" on an all-women's locked ward. At first, because I grew up with all of the stereotypes about "mental patients," I had trouble distinguishing the patients from the nurses. Of the thirty or forty women on my ward, only one or two looked like those stereotypes. As we listened to one another's stories, a picture of how sexism had led to each of us being there emerged, but it was not until many years later, after learning how sexism and mental health oppression intertwine, that I realized it.

One young woman, aged 16, had been raped by her brother-in-law and got pretty scared as a result. In the hospital she was given electroshock, which terrified her even more. Another woman was depressed because her husband beat her. He then had her committed for depression. A few women were there because they couldn't figure out what they wanted to do

---

* This article uses the term *mentalism* to refer to the kind of oppression that people put on other people when they expect them to think a certain way.

with their lives. Two or three others were lesbians, which was considered "mentally ill."

After leaving the hospital, I continued to hear the same kinds of stories from other ex-patients. One woman suffered from exhaustion while trying to raise several young children, one of whom woke up screaming half of the night. She was also dealing with a husband who wouldn't take any responsibility for the children and who blamed all of the difficulties on her. She was given psychotropic drugs to deal with the fact that she cried a lot. Another woman was depressed about a miscarriage she'd had; this led to a series of commitments. A third woman was sexually abused but did not remember it until years later. When the feelings started to surface, she thought she was going crazy. Another young woman, alone and trying to care for her mother who was dying from cancer, began to have thoughts about life and death. She was committed by her father for having these thoughts. Her "therapy" consisted of having her long hair pulled by her psychiatrist whenever she voiced her thoughts on the subject. She also had a series of electroshocks which, after twenty years, she still has nightmares about. She was pronounced cured when she no longer voiced the thoughts (though she still had them after all of her "treatments"). A very large woman was committed for being "too" loud and aggressive. A college student, concerned about ending racism rather than about getting dates, was considered crazy and got a series of electroshocks and several "hospitalizations."

The underlying theme in all of these stories is that the women had problems because of sexism. Instead of society addressing the sexism, the women were further victimized by having their difficulties medicalized, making it appear that there was something wrong with *them*. This is commonly known as "blaming the victim." How and why does this happen? To answer that question, we have to take a look at how mentalism works in general and then consider how it intertwines with other oppressions, particularly sexism.

Definition of Mentalism

What is mentalism? It's the weaning away of ourselves from ourselves; the enforcement of who we are "supposed to be" instead of who we are; the glorification of pretense and the denial of our humanness. It is the denial of our abilities to perceive, think, decide, act, feel, and release emotions. It is the denial of our ability to understand ourselves in new ways and to change our lives and our world. It's a big "Go to your room until you can behave" sign, and in this case your room is the "mental hospital." It is the manufacturing of conformity, of the status quo, of so-called "normality" into what is called "reality."

If people don't like being the victims of oppression, they are told, "That's just the way it is. You can't fight city hall." We are expected to believe that people can't really change, that their distresses are natural and inherent, that "boys will be boys," that sexism is biological. Stepping outside our socially conditioned roles and thinking differently is called "crazy." The idea that you can lose your mind, that it is not permanently yours, that it can become unavailable to you in ways other than physical brain damage, permeates our society. Most people tend to fear "going crazy" and/or doubt or mistrust their own thinking as a result of this oppression. These beliefs are institutionalized in the "mental health" and other systems, notably the school and the legal systems.

Foundations of Oppression

The foundations of mentalism begin with very young babies as their parents and/or other adult caretakers stop their natural emotional release and healing processes and enforce the "way to be."* Parents and other caretakers tend to re-enact with children how they themselves were punished, scolded, ignored, humiliated, etc. The children therefore become conditioned to stop running; playing; snuggling; being loud, joyful, enthusiastic, spontaneous, or silly; and even talking. When was the last time you, as an adult, were moved to do some of those

---

* This is not intended as a putdown of parents or other adults. I am a parent myself, so I understand how hard it can be to listen to a crying baby while you yourself are falling asleep in the middle of the night, or trying to make dinner or get to work on time. Equally hard is to allow your child to cry and scream in a restaurant in the middle of a meal. Parents in our society do not have the support needed to really listen at length to children, nor is our society set up to deal with children's or adults' emotional needs. Parents are put in the unenviable position of having to "control" their children's emotions and actions so that they will conform to society's "norms."

things, did so without embarrassment or discomfort, or did so at all? In school, all of this prohibition of natural human responses is reinforced. Furthermore, students are divided along classist, racist, sexist, and ableist lines. If one does not conform to these divisions, one is not acceptable.

A child with difficulties becomes a "problem" student with "dyslexia," "hyperactivity," "attention deficit," "conduct disorder," or some other classified problem. Such students are put into "emotionally disturbed" classes and usually stay there. Many are forced to take drugs, most commonly Ritalin. Children who continue to be rebellious, "different," end up in the "mental health" system, reform school, and other institutions. As a teen or young adult, the squeeze comes: Be adult or else. Many of us had our first experiences with the mental health system at that age because the pressure to fit into society's roles becomes intense at that point. We believe that we aren't good enough, smart enough, OK enough, can't get real help, can't be close, and we keep our stories to ourselves as we take on our adult roles.

How Mentalism Works

In one sense, mentalism is not about mental patients and hospitals but about their use as symbols to control the whole society. "Mental patients" are the butt end of classism. Somebody has to be poor for capitalism to work, and it's the "defectives" who are most OK to be those people. They are the ultimate scapegoat and the excuse for not looking at what's wrong with our society. If people cannot function in the ways they are supposed to, hold down a job, or behave in socially acceptable ways; if they can't be "cured" to do that, it's their fault, so the "reasoning" goes, and we don't have to look at the racism, classism, sexism, and so on that put them at the bottom of the society in the first place. We also don't have to look at our own distress because *they* are the problem, not us.

To have a society based on making money at all costs instead of on people and their real needs, you have to denigrate and punish things like caring, needing help, and all of the emotional healing processes; otherwise, people will not stay lock-step in the roles required to keep the oppressive society going. If people are allowed and encouraged to heal themselves emotionally, they begin to stop numbing out with addictions and become more aware. They begin to question injustice and fight oppression.

Mentalism puts a damper on spontaneity, creativity, and any kind of "differentness," including that of oppressed groups. What society calls "normality" is the average of the ways the dominant oppressor group has been socialized into behaving—the ways white, adult, male, heterosexual, able-bodied, Anglo-Saxon, Protestant, middle- or owning-class people are supposed to behave. Not that there is necessarily something wrong with being a member of those groups, but the stereotypes of how they are "supposed to be," the ways into which they are often smashed into behaving, are the standards by which everyone else's behavior is judged. They determine the "most acceptable" ways to act, and these become the ones most people are comfortable with because society promotes them as "normal." These behaviors are not recognized as being acquired, rigid, or socially conditioned. They are what I call "chronically normal" behavior patterns.

Oppressed groups are allowed their uniqueness but only if they agree that these traits are not OK. For example, artists can create but are crazy, women can cry but are hysterical, and so on. In general, mentalism takes any human quality that is not useful for maintaining oppression, and puts it down.

Mentalism is the stop sign on all liberation efforts. People who step outside their designated oppressor or oppressed roles are called "crazy," officially or unofficially. This oppression also stops us from reclaiming our power and feeling hopeful. There is a terror of functioning "way out there," very powerfully. It means that acting from your true nature, aware and fully empowered, may make you appear "crazy" to others and even feel "crazy" to yourself. Some of us were actually reclaiming some of our power when we were labeled.

Mentalism intertwines with other key oppressions:

▲ *Racism and antisemitism.* The "defect theory" suggests that certain groups of people are biologically inferior, or dangerous to society, or both, and should be eliminated. This was promoted by the eugenics movement during the height of Nazi power in the 1930s and 1940s. Psychiatrists were some of the main theorists of that movement and had thousands of mental patients killed in the forerunner of the Holocaust. Biogenetic theories in psychiatry today are mainstream and support the new racist "violence initiative" by the U.S. National Institute of Mental Health under the National Institute of Health, the Department of Justice, the National Science Foundation, and the Center for Disease Control to locate children in the inner cities of the U.S. (i.e. primarily people of color) who are "predisposed to violence" and drug them in order to "cure" them.[*]

▲ *Oppression of physically disabled people.* Like psychiatric survivors, disabled people are considered useless to society due to their supposed inability to produce economic goods. As a result, they are isolated from public view and are often put into institutions very similar to mental hospitals. They are disempowered and mistreated in the medical system and shunned by the larger society the same way that psychiatric survivors are—as if they can't think for themselves or make their own decisions, as if they are "weird" or even "crazy." Real physical problems are often considered to be "mental problems"; it is not considered normal to have a physical disability. Rather than recognizing that everyone's physical nature is fine with all of our "imperfections," and that society needs to take into account all of these differences, the supposedly "able-bodied" hide and deny their physical difficulties for fear of being labeled and rejected, and disabled people are made to feel out of step.

▲ *Gay and lesbian oppression.* Despite being officially not "ill," according to the latest revised psychiatric diagnostic manual, in practice gays and lesbians are still often treated as if mentally ill. Even stepping outside of gender roles, regardless of whether or not one is gay or lesbian, is enough to be labeled "crazy."

▲ *Sexism.* The oppression of women reinforces the general demeaning of emotions, emotional release, and vulnerability, and promotes the worship of individuality and competition. The mental health system is, in one sense, the institutionalization of sexism and homophobia.

---

[*] This project is currently in the research stages and is further described in Dr. Peter Breggin, *The War Against Children* (New York: St. Martin's, 1994).

What is "Mental Illness"?

If you understand how oppression works and how the natural healing processes work, you can see that there is no such thing as mental illness, being crazy, insane, nuts, off your rocker, and so on. What people call "mental illness" is usually someone's attempt to use the natural emotional release healing process. The attempt is sometimes productive but is often misinterpreted and cut off by others. The notion of "mental illness" is a fabrication designed to keep us from our real selves and to keep us from ending oppression. There is no "normal," no line that separates "crazy" people from "sane" people.

So how do we get separated from the general population? Certain ways we've been hurt (and then tend to re-enact the hurt on ourselves and others) are seen as "not OK"; others are "OK." Most people act "chronically normal"—"this is the way it is"—based on classism. Oppressor and oppressed roles are "normal," and "normal" is defined differently in different cultures. In U.S. culture, "OK" ways to act out how we got hurt include building bombs, spending money on warfare rather than on things people need, competing when cooperating would make more sense, being "cool," being distant, smoking, social drinking, yelling at children, and pretending to feel fine all the time while hurting deeply, to name a few. Yet most of these behaviors are "dangerous to self or others" (part of the standard for committing people to mental hospitals). It is not "OK" to stay in bed all day, or to rage, shake, tremble, or even laugh loudly in public. While it is "OK" to kill yourself by smoking excessively, driving dangerously, or overworking, it is not "OK" to do so by taking an overdose of pills or jumping out a window. Once you've been labeled, almost anything can be seen as inappropriate—people have literally been rehospitalized for sleeping on the couch, eating a cold dinner on the porch, or wearing too many coats!

People usually get labeled "mentally ill" for crying, raging, or otherwise releasing emotions "too much," or for attempting to get to the emotional release by re-enacting some or all of how they were hurt in the first place, in the hopes of getting help with it. This natural healing process is called "strange," "sick," and "incomprehensible."

What is a "nervous breakdown"? It's usually *lots* of emotional release. Rigidly conditioned behavior, often the behavior that holds the emotions tightly in check, is what is breaking down, not the nerves.

What are hallucinations and "delusions"? Hallucinations naturally occur when a person has accumulated so much distress that his or her physical survival is threatened and at the same time he or she has so many inhibitions as to make emotional release virtually impossible. At this point, the person sees and/or hears whatever will allow the emotional release and healing to begin, i.e. "clues" to what the person needs to laugh, shake, or cry about. "Delusions" are logical conclusions based on incorrect assumptions and/or feelings from old hurts that appear to be occurring in the present.

What are some other reasons people get labeled? Spiritual experiences may provide insights useful to the person and/or society, but people who have them tend to be labeled "mentally ill." A child trying desperately to counsel the family in order to help the parents get back on track so that they can parent well is declared "mentally ill."

My favorite story is about a feminist author who tells about how she gave a lot of money to help get an African anti-apartheid leader out of jail in South Africa. To her family of white U.S.'ers, this was stepping outside the roles created for them by racism. To them, she was acting "crazy," and she ended up in a mental hospital as a result.

In the U.S., it used to be immigrants who were put in institutions; now it is homeless people. Occasionally physical diseases such as Alzheimer's, syphilis, brain tumors, nutritional deficiency, or chemical sensitivity can be what leads to being labeled, but these are much rarer than the usual situation of overload of distress and can be detected through medical tests.

None of these situations, in any case, is helped by psychiatric drugs or other punishments. The biological/genetic theories of mental illness are unfounded and unproven, yet they continue to be accepted as fact by most people. They are used to promote billions in profits for the drug companies, which, incidentally, made more money than the oil companies last year in 1992. There is no price regulation of drug sales in the U.S.; the "war on drugs" excludes the government-sponsored ones. The newer moneymaking industry is shock treatment. Psychiatric drugs and shock are creating a new category of brain-damaged people who tend to stay in the mental health system permanently as "outpatients." Now psychiatrists can "prove" we have "different" brains because of the damage caused by drugs and shock.

Sexism and Mentalism

What part does all of this play in keeping women from achieving equal status in the society? It plays a big one. The majority of patients in the mental health system are women, and the majority of patients in the mental health system receiving electroshock and being prescribed psychiatric drugs are women. The natural processes that women have stayed in touch with, processes that are considered to be too "feminine" for men, such as crying or talking about feelings and releasing them, are labeled as *symptoms*.

The mental health system is, in many ways, the institutionalization of sexism. Here the doctor's word is law, and the vast majority of psychiatrists, certainly nearly all of the senior ones, are male. They are at the top of a very rigid hierarchy. Patients, most of whom are either women or men who are looked upon as victimized sissies who cannot fulfill the male role (or seen as "violent animals"), are at the very bottom of the hierarchy. Psychiatric technicians, social workers, and nurses, virtually all female, must kowtow to the doctors. The entire system reinforces the sexist mainstream societal views of men and women.

Mental health workers must act normal, i.e. the way men are supposed to act. They must always appear in charge, know all of the answers, analyze rather than feel or use intuition, and resist showing any emotion or feeling. Above all, they must never have problems themselves. On the one hand, they must be "professional," distant, and avoid close physical or emotional contact with their patients. On the other hand, male psychiatrists and other therapists can easily, in secret, sexually exploit and abuse their female patients with little or no fear of punishment.

Power imbalance makes the abuse easy. Psychiatrists can commit people to psychiatric institutions without due process. They can force people to take brain-damaging drugs with no questions asked. And "therapy" is always a one-way street. The therapist can never admit to having problems.

Because women are conditioned by sexism to be victims, they tend to go along with whatever the therapist says—"Doctor knows best." If they don't, their protests can always be silenced with drugs, electroshock, solitary confinement or having what they say invalidated because, after all, they are the ones labeled "crazy," not the "therapists."

The natural healing process requires warm, physical and emotional (but nonsexual) closeness, similar to the way babies heal themselves in their mothers' arms. It also requires vulnerability and lots of emotional release. Many women are in touch with these things, but this kind of behavior, for adults, is invalidated by the system and labeled as symptomatic of mental illness. Women are pronounced mentally healthy when they have learned to hold things in, not to be vulnerable, not to ask for help, not to appear needy, and to act out the "feminine" roles of returning to their husbands, getting back to housework and child care, getting married, dating men, and so on.

Being a lesbian or bisexual woman is not considered mentally healthy; and the "normal" sexual orientation, which puts women in the role of passive sex object, pleasing the man no matter what she really wants, and puts men in the role of individuals with massive, uncontrollable sex drive, is never questioned.

Rugged independence and competitiveness are considered mentally healthy. They are encouraged by the rigid hierarchy of the system, even down to the hospital wards where one moves to less and less restricted areas based on "good behavior" and often by supervising other patients, under the eye of the psychiatric technician or nurse, of course. Patients are endlessly compared to one another as to who is the most "sick." Fraternizing "too much" with other patients or patients helping each other is considered dangerous and is discouraged. Patients' governments, councils, and so on are usually in name only.

Proposals for Change

What can be done about this situation? Where do we go from here? The most basic thing we women psychiatric survivors need to do is make friends and form alliances with other women, particularly those who are active in the women's movement. We need to become more active and visible in it ourselves. For many of us, because we have stepped outside of female roles and therefore been labeled "crazy" or "unfeminine," it feels hard to identify with other women. It is important to go against those feelings and join with our sisters, for our own sake as well as theirs. Battered women, sexual abuse survivors, rape victims, and others have many issues in common with us and are our natural allies. Our issues are important for all women because mentalism acts as a threat to all women. Women's liberation cannot be achieved without taking these issues into account. Beyond that basic aligning of ourselves with the women's movement, we must do other important work:

▲ *We must reclaim our inherent power.* When I say power, I don't mean the false idea of power we've been given by our society—as in, the person with the most power dominates the most people, kills the most people with the most weapons, and so on—and I'm not talking about physical power (though for most women who have been denied this, it's a good idea to reclaim some of it). I'm talking about the kind of power that stimulates and nurtures emotional growth; that organizes people to bridge cultural, racial, and other barriers; that organizes people to fight for and gain their rights; that promotes people making things right in the society; that helps people to heal themselves, each other, and the environment. True power promotes equality, justice, caring, and cooperation among all people; it seeks to lead people to lead other people to do the same and does not ask anyone to become a mechanized follower.

One way I've reclaimed my own power is to speak out whenever and wherever I get a chance about our issues. I try to make allies as I speak rather than speaking from a position of anger. I tell people how this issue affects *everyone* personally and invite them to join us. When I was institutionalized, I was locked in "seclusion" for many hours. As a woman who had already been very intimidated by my experiences with sexism, I became even more submissive, quiet, and accommodating as a result. Speaking out against this was hard for me at first. I had to break through the ways I'd been conditioned to be silent. Now it is easy for me to speak out and it has become fun as well.

Speaking out was the first step toward reclaiming my power, and it led to many others. About three years after first speaking out, I made a decision that totally changed my life and career. I decided to see that mentalism is ended. In order to do that, I had to stop being a full-time visual artist and become a full-time mental health liberation leader, which I now am. If anyone had told me fifteen years ago that I could create my own career in a field that was pretty much nonexistent, I would not have believed it. The decision, which I stuck to, led me to many powerful possibilities. It took ten years, but I am now doing work I love, leading workshops on reclaiming power and natural healing processes; coordinating survivors' conferences; and co-coordinating Support Coalition International, a coalition for human rights and alternatives to psychiatry. Other women can make the same decision; here's how: First, practice deciding it aloud, preferably with a friend who is listening supportively: "From now on I am completely in charge of mental health liberation and I decide to end oppression. And this means . . . [whatever it means to you]." Say whatever your thought is, even if it makes no sense. Eventually you'll start saying things that you would do if you knew you were in charge. (If not each of us, then who's in charge of our liberation?) When you are ready, try making the decision as a real decision and actually do the things you thought of (the ones that make sense, of course). Each beginning action, however insignificant, will lead you to the next step.

Doing anything against the oppression, no matter what it is, begins to destroy powerlessness and leads to reclaiming more power. We can reclaim our power in many areas: in our ability to heal ourselves and nurture others to do the same; to make our personal lives go well; to create safe, healing environments; to organize for social change among ourselves and in coalition with other movements; and more. There are no limits to what we can do in the long run, though there may be obstacles to surmount in the short run.

Another decision that can help us reclaim power is "From now on, I fiercely decide to never again settle for anything less than ABSOLUTELY EVERYTHING! and that means . . ."

▲ *We must create women psychiatric survivors' support groups and other women's support groups.* It is easier for us to tell our stories and heal with people we feel connected to, i.e., those with stories similar to ours. In the long run, we need to reclaim our unity with all people so that we don't remain separated, but it is important first to build unity with those who are most like us.

In my experience, the most workable way to run such a group is to give each woman equal time to talk about whatever she wants to while others in the group listen attentively and caringly, without comments, positive or negative, and without advice or interruption of any kind. The space to be listened to allows each woman to trust her own thinking, to take charge of her own life. If advice and comments are offered, people are reminded of group therapy. Allowing each woman an equal amount of time to talk is important in order to avoid having talkative people dominate the group. In the case of someone who feels she hasn't much to say, it's fine if she gets listened to anyway, even if some or most of her time is spent in silence. Eventually she will feel safe enough to talk. Confidentiality is also important, especially if the women see each other outside of the group; it's important not to bring up things discussed in the group, unless the person herself brings it up or gives her permission for others to do so. Finally, groups should be small. When there are eight or so members in the group and others want to join, start another group so that it doesn't get too large and unwieldy.

Leaders' groups for leaders of women survivors' groups can be held periodically to bring leaders together to share thinking and support. It works well to have each woman take an equal amount of time to answer the following questions: What's the current situation for women psychiatric survivors (locally, nationally, internationally)? How have I recently contributed to our liberation efforts? What is my next step in leading toward our liberation? What could hold me back from that step? How am I going to surmount what could hold me back? What kinds of support could I use from those here in surmounting the obstacles? Set up specific support then and there, if possible.

▲ *We must create personal support systems and other alternatives.* There is no way that I could keep going with all of the liberation work I do without my support network. I would have burned out long ago. Every week I spend three hours exchanging listening/healing time (1.5 hours each) with a close friend with whom I've been doing this for fifteen years. Though he is male and not a psychiatric survivor, he understands my issues well and speaks out about them publicly—he's a great ally. We tend to each do a lot of sobbing when being listened to by the other. This always clears my thinking, gets my mind off of my problems, and helps me to refocus on my goals. I also have shorter listening times with four women locally (each once a month) and occasional time with about ten or twelve psychiatric survivor leaders across the country. In addition, I meet bimonthly with ten psychiatric survivor leaders in a regional support group, and about every six months I hold a leaders' meeting as described above with survivor leaders from Pennsylvania and New Jersey. I stay in touch by phone and letter with many survivor leaders, especially those involved in Support Coalition International. As co-coordinators of that coalition, David Oakes and I talk every week on the phone. Whenever I go to a mental health conference, especially one for survivors, I do a workshop on supporting each other and meet more people interested in being part of the network. Some of us hold both formal and informal support groups at free times during the conference. (That's how I get through conferences without getting overwhelmed and worn out.)

I used to get very depressed and feel completely alone and unable to call for help. Now there are so many people I can call when I start to feel that way that it never lasts for more than a few minutes. I think everyone, but especially psychiatric survivor leaders ought to create a support system for themselves similar to this one. The oppression we are fighting is extremely vicious and if we are to keep going, we will need all the support we can get. Also, when we support each other, we help put psychiatry out of business.

Part of my vision for ending psychiatric oppression is to create so many survivor-run support systems that work well that the mental health system as we know it today withers away for lack of use, replaced by a humane network of caring people.

Other kinds of alternatives that need to be created are safe houses (residences that provide child care and other supports for people in crisis), survivor-run apartment complexes (like the Community For Interdependent Living, which is run by one of our coalition group members in San Jose, CA), detox centers for people who want to get off psychiatric drugs safely, cooperative living communities, and organizations that promote the arts and do advocacy at the same time (like Altered States of the Arts, another group in our coalition). Many more alternative groups that we haven't even thought of yet will be created in the years ahead.

▲ *We must organize in coalitions for social change.* We need to organize ourselves so that we have enough political clout to make an impact. The larger, more unified and more inclusive our organizations are, the more political influence we will have. If we organize around broad issues that are important to everyone, including survivor subgroups, such as survivors of color, elder survivors, physically disabled survivors, young survivors, and so on, we will be more effective by promoting unity.*

There is much that can be done to fight our double oppression as women psychiatric survivors. I am increasingly excited about the possibilities.

---

* For information about how you or your group can join Support Coalition International, please write to Janet Foner at 920 Brandt Ave., New Cumberland, PA 17070.

HOW TO RESPOND TO YOUR PSYCHIATRICALLY LABELED FRIEND OR RELATIVE

(who may appear "mad" or in a trance-like state)

Victoria Papers

1. Realize that they are not "mentally ill" but they can be made mentally ill by the reactions and misunderstandings of others.

2. Realize that there are different levels of reality—even going into a trancelike state is within the range of what should be considered normal human experience.

3. Realize that they have a special gift—a genetic endowment that increases creativity and perceptions of reality. Don't try to stifle it—you will just cause added pressure.

4. If your friend or relative does go into a trancelike state, DO NOT TAKE THEM TO THE MENTAL HEALTH RESOURCE CENTER OR ANY PSYCHIATRIC WARD. This is extremely important. Being in unfamiliar surroundings among strangers in this trancelike dream state is very frightening—as a horror nightmare. In fear they may cry out or attack, and then they will likely be put in the lock-up room tied hand and foot to the bed for hours. If you have done this to your friend or relative, go lie on your bed and put your hands and feet as though they were tied up—imagine staying that way without being able to

move for hours. DEAL WITH YOUR OWN LACK OF COMPASSION AND SELFISHNESS!

5. DO NOT TAKE THEM FOR DELIVERANCE TO CAST THE DEVIL OUT! What people have done in their ignorance is deplorable!

6. Protect them from people who do not understand.

7. Do not probe them and incite them.

8. Do not get out a tape recorder and record their seemingly irrational dreamlike statements to play for others later. (Yes, people have done that!)

9. Do not call them crazy.

10. Respond to them calmly and respectfully. If not incited, they will usually go to sleep. Much of what they are doing is talking in their sleep.

11. Playing soft music may be helpful. Assure them of love and caring and that they are in a safe place and among people they can trust and who love them. You might read them comforting words.

12. Realize that what they say is dreamlike-symbolic and may have meaning totally the opposite of what the seeing eye or hearing ear would judge it to be.

13. Treat them with respect. When they return to the conscious state, don't call them crazy, or mock what they said while in the subconscious state. Listen to their explanation of what they feel they experienced. Learn from them.

14. Treat the whole situation as normal because it is!

15. Realize that there is a difference between a nervous breakdown and a spiritual experience.

16. Realize that every person's experience is individual and you need wisdom to discern each situation.

I have gone into a trancelike state a number of times and I have written out this list of what I feel should be done for me.

MADWOMAN

Elaine Erickson

Love is so far away,
like sea gulls circling into the past.

She digs into the dirt of her plants, wild flowers
flowing from her fingers.

Swept aside because she can no longer
be believed, she ascends

the stairs to the attic,
her cries echoing down a stairwell.

And who are her oppressors? Do they sit in their trucks,
dialing an oath for her on the phone?

Or do they hug their knees
and sweat from her passionate gaze?

She only knows they are relentless,
these voices that nail her to every word she speaks.

She's one hell of a human being, you know, they tell her,
a whore and an old maid in one

and when she's done
crying out her life

she'll descend to the cellar
and wait to hear one far-away bird

cry with hope.

TESTIMONY*

Lorelee Stewart

My name is Lorelee Stewart. I live in Revere, Massachusetts. I am a 27-year-old Personal Assistance Services user with a psychiatric disability. I am the External Vice President of the National Council on Independent Living and a member of the National Association of Psychiatric Survivors. I'm very honored to be here today to testify on the need for a National Personal Assistance Services Program, which among other groups would serve people with psychiatric disabilities. I commend Senator Kennedy and the other committee members for their foresight in holding this hearing to illuminate and document the national need for Personal Assistance Services.

I currently work as the Executive Director of the Independent Living Center of the North Shore, a human service agency which helps disabled people live independently in the community with appropriate support services. Our center is run and staffed by disabled people, and we are all given Reasonable Accommodation to do our jobs. For me, part of my Reasonable Accommodation is to receive Personal Assistance Services when needed for job-related activities. Primarily, I use this assistance for traveling. This is paid for by my employer. My employment situation is unfortunately rare. Normally, disabled people who need Personal Assistance Services are only given them as a work accommodation from organizations that are run by other

---

* Testimony of Lorelee Stewart Before the Senate Labor and Human Resources Committee Regarding Personal Assistance Services, July 25, 1991.

disabled people. I am not eligible for the Massachusetts Personal Care Assistance Program, which is run through Medicaid, because of its categorical approach to eligibility, which excludes my disability.

I became disabled at the tender age of four when two uncles began to sadistically abuse me, physically, mentally, and sexually. This continued for over fourteen years. Life for me is a daily struggle. The after effects of this prolonged abuse have caused my psychiatric condition, which is Chronic Post Traumatic Stress Disorder, a condition made famous by the Vietnam veterans.

I didn't remember my childhood at all until I was twenty. I felt empty and asleep. Then one day during my junior year at Harvard College, I woke up, alive and hurting. I began to have flashbacks of the abuse. I basically have four types of flashbacks: a scene flashback, where I see pictures of the abuse as if I were reliving it without the feelings; a feeling flashback, or a panic attack, where I have no mental pictures of the abuse but experience the fear and terror of the abusive acts; a sensory flashback, which contains no pictures or feelings but may have smells or sounds that were part of the acts, like commands, screams, cologne, or alcohol; or a complete flashback where all or some of these sensations are combined into a more total and frightening picture of the abuse.

At times I feel extremely depressed and suicidal, wishing I had never survived the abuse at all. This, I'm told, is very common for abuse survivors. I also have a sleep disorder and additional physical illnesses as a result of the extreme stress I live with.

These disabling effects make it difficult at times to perform simple activities of daily living. There are times when I am completely capable of handling everything. There are also times when, due to my disability, I barely get by and need a lot of assistance. With the exception of work, this help comes from family and friends, often placing strains on my personal relationships and prematurely ending some friendships simply because the help I needed had become too much of a burden. I feel that this level of assistance is beyond what should be expected of a friend or family member.

I would like to be able to pay an assistant to do the things that my friends do now, begrudgingly, for free. I do have a psychiatrist and a psychologist that I work with. They, of course, are both paid. I use them for specific things that require extensive training like psychopharmacology and 24-hour emergency crisis link-up. Most of the help that I need does not require the same degree of expertise and training. I have people who help me balance my checkbook when I cannot do so myself because I'm depressed and people who accompany me on a food shopping trip because I feel too panicked to go alone, for fear I might have a flashback in public. Many times, I pay $8-$10 an hour for someone to assist me in these ways. When I cannot find a volunteer or don't have the money to hire someone, I go without help and my ability to do things is limited and my safety becomes endangered.

Having this type of assistance enables me to follow the advice of my doctors even when my panic attacks are so severe that I cannot remember to take my medicine. The best analogy I can make is someone who, when they're healthy, designs a living will or a Health Care Proxy to make decisions for themselves when they become unable to do so. When I ask someone to work for me, I teach them how to do things that I temporarily cannot do for myself. In the event of a severe panic attack, my assistant, who has been previously trained by me to give me my prescribed dosage, does so and I eventually feel better. If I don't have this type of assistance, the only other option is hospitalization or a day treatment program. Neither of these options allow me to maintain a job. I would like to reiterate that the assistance I need is due to a disability and is not the result of laziness. A personal assistant is by no means a maid service.

I would like to see a National Personal Assistance Services Program set up that has eligibility criteria that are based on functional limitation rather than disability label. People with all types of disabilities can benefit from some kind of Personal Assistance Services. Because I am involved on the national level with many people who have psychiatric disabilities, I am certain that others will want to use Personal Assistance Services to help them live more independent fulfilling lives. The philosophy that is used for Personal Assistance Services for persons with physical disabilities would work equally well for people with psychiatric disabilities. Essentially, assistance provided by an employee of the disabled person performs tasks the disabled person can't do because of their disability. This provides dignity, control, and independence. Consumer control has been the key to successful

Personal Assistance Services for people with physical disabilities and would be so for a program that included psychiatric disabilities as well. People with psychiatric disabilities do not want to be assigned a "caretaker" to watch over them paternalistically. We want to have complete control over who assists us with our personal matters.

Drastic policy changes need to be made in this country in order for disabled persons to truly take their place in society as independent, productive citizens. The Americans with Disabilities Act has explicitly promised this to the disability community. However, without a comprehensive, cross-disability, consumer-controlled Personal Assistance Services program and other necessary community-oriented assistance, the dream of the Americans with Disabilities Act will never be fulfilled. Those who are most severely disabled, yet able to live and work independently with Personal Assistance Services, will be left behind as unnecessary prisoners of institutions without them.

The concept of Personal Assistance Services is truly beautiful because it makes all policymakers happy. If you are concerned with establishing policy that ensures people's civil rights, and gives them independence and dignity, Personal Assistance Services is the way to go.

If you are a policymaker who is concerned with a service system that has proven success and is cost effective, then a Personal Assistance Services Program is the way to go. Personal Assistance Services makes everyone a winner: the policymakers, the independent individuals with disabilities, and the society that benefits from their presence.

Again, thank you for the opportunity to speak before you today on the need for a National Personal Assistance Program. I look forward to supporting your efforts in any way possible.

MOVING OUT OF ISOLATION

Kris Yates

The challenge of feeling close and connected to others is something that I struggle with in my life. On the surface, I am a warm, friendly person, and most folks would never dream how alone I often feel. It is particularly difficult for me to show others my neediness and pain. I have a strong pattern of making sure I "look good." Although this pattern probably began in early childhood when I lived alone with my mother and there was no help available, my experience with the mental health system has only strengthened the pattern.

Looking "good" feels like insurance against getting locked up. Of course, it is no insurance at all, because it is often after years of "holding it together" that feelings just pop out and everything goes out of control. That's sort of what happened to me in India when I got put in the Hospital for Mental Diseases. It was there that I had the worst experiences of my life: ECT, forced drugging, and seclusion. These things alone make it hard for me to know that I can get close to others.

What is done to us by the mental health system when we are in need of connection and human contact is horrendous. When I was really hurting, I was put in isolation, drugged, and given a stigma which carries the message that I am a defective human being, "abnormal." This experience gave me an invisible suitcase of shame that I carry with me wherever I go. The experience of being separated from other people when I was severely hurting translates into "Don't let anyone know how bad it is or you will be left alone."

When I returned from India to the U.S., I was met at the airport by an official from the U.S. Department of Health, Education and Welfare. I told him that I wanted to see an acupuncturist, and he responded by saying he would take me to a "doctor"; he then proceeded to take me to a locked psychiatric ward. As soon as I realized where I was being taken, I became hysterical (a normal healthy response, in my opinion, given that I had just returned from being hospitalized against my will and received "treatment" in the form of ECT). As a result, I was put in restraints and placed in seclusion.

What's the message I got? Don't show your feelings. Keep feelings under control. If you show your feelings, you will be separated from other people. Don't let anyone know what is really going on inside of you, or you will be punished.

I'm thinking about how, when I am crying really hard and someone moves in physically close to me, I immediately stop crying. I always assumed my response had something to do with having a domineering, suffocating mother and that if I didn't have a certain amount of physical space, it felt like my mother moving in on me. Now I am wondering if this reaction isn't also connected to having been held down and drugged when I was upset in the hospital.

It is horrible to be forcibly held down and have needles jabbed into your arms or buttocks. When I left the hospital in India, I had knots four inches in diameter in both arms and buttocks from needles—testimony to my struggles against their weapons. And who won the fight? I guess I did because I am now out and free. But while I was there I stopped fighting because their weapons were too powerful.

Now the challenge is to get the fight back and to realize that it is not only safe but crucial that I get close to other people. My continued growth and flourishing depends on my reclaiming the parts of me that almost got crushed by the hospital. The "almost" part is very important because I know that I am still whole and able to completely heal in spite of all they did.

There was also a strong message in the hospital that "Fighting gets you nowhere." While I was there, I fought with everything I had and I got hurt for it. Never in my life had I fought so hard. Now I want to recover from the message to "keep everything under control." In order to live my life fully, I must have my passion and rage. Otherwise, I simply "settle" for whatever comes my way. The enforced passivity I received in the hospital was very damaging. I must transcend that passivity, particularly as a woman, in order to really live.

The challenge for me is to reclaim that fight and apply it toward making my life all that it can be, getting what I deserve, and seeking justice in the ways that are closest to my heart. The challenge is also to know that I am lovable, capable of complete intimacy, and naturally connected to others. Young children demonstrate their knowledge of connection by the way they eagerly go after other children, adults, and animals. I also want to learn that I can show my real hurts to others and no one will go away, and I won't be taken away. Looking "good" has served its purpose and is always available to me if I need it. But now it's time I let the guard down in order to let others in. That pattern has served its purpose and can move over to let the vulnerable me show.

WORKING THE SYSTEM

Anne C. Woodlen

I have been involved with the mental health system for thirty-three years, and I want to share with you what I've experienced as a worker in the system.

About twenty years ago, I suffered major psychiatric hospitalizations. After that spell of troubles had abated, I went to Vocational and Educational Services for Individuals with Disabilities (VESID)—it was the Office of Vocational Rehabilitation (OVR) in those days—and went through a lot of professional testing that told me what I already knew: I was gifted and should do something significant with my life. OVR sent me to Syracuse University, but I dropped out after one semester.

For most of my adult life, I have been employed in a variety of jobs that didn't fit. I got fired a lot but hung onto marginal employment by working as a temporary employee for many years. I got my own version of a liberal arts education.

About eight years ago, I went to work for a friend in the mental health system; I became an administrative assistant in the regional Office of Mental Health. When I was hospitalized again during the course of that employment, the system's response was to try to fire me. The regional director went to bat for me; he was quoted as saying, "If we can't take care of our own, then what the hell good are we?" My job was saved for the moment, but three years later I was fired by a person who was insensitive to the disabilities I was working with.

I went back to OVR and they sent me back to school, this time to a community college. After nearly two years there, I got an associate's degree, but then had to drop away from my goal of a master's degree because I was quite ill from the side effects of psychiatric medication.

Several years ago, at a time when I was homeless, I got connected with the Transitional Living Service (TLS). I lived in one of their supported apartments and worked with a case manager. The case manager routinely kept me informed about various job preparation activities that TLS held. One in particular that stood out in my mind was a course called Self-Directed Rehabilitation that was taught by a dreamer from New York City and a consumer from the Mental Health Association. We were invited to dream about our own futures, and I ended up being able to say, "I am a writer; I have been a writer all my life but now I want to become a *published* writer."

I needed some structure—a context within which to work—and TLS provided it. Their aptly-named support center was the place where I hung my hat and worked at writing. There was an informal support structure that encouraged me. One of the things I did was publish the first issue of my own newsletter.

One of the more specific supports that TLS provided was a job group. It was composed of recipients of mental health services who stood in some relation to work: trying to choose a career, get an education for a career, get a job, keep a job, figure out why you lost a job. Some fifteen or twenty people went through the group while I was there; many stopped coming because they got full-time employment. It was a place where we could celebrate with each other in success and learn in failure. Not insignificantly, it was also a place where we could share the hard facts of how working affects Medicaid, SSI, Disability, and other aspects of the system.

It was with the support of the job group that I went back to work part-time as a companion to elderly women. Also, I became a staff writer for a newsletter published by the Mental Health Association. Then, as a result of the newsletter I published, I came in contact with the Mental Patients' Liberation Alliance and I was invited to apply for part-time work as an administrative assistant. I knew that my commitment was to becoming a published writer, but I also knew that I needed a "day job," so I went to work for the Alliance.

One of the things I identified in working with TLS was that it is important to me to have a job to which I can make a moral commitment; a job where I can see an ideal and work to make it real. The Office of Mental Health was not such a place; the

Alliance is. At the Alliance we want nothing less than freedom and empowerment for all people. I care about that, and so, in the daily business of the empowerment movement, I do data entry, prepare speeches, assist in mailings, and generally keep things tucked in and properly organized. Two months ago I became a full-time administrative assistant for the Alliance.

I've reached the conclusion that OVR wasted a lot of money sending me to school because all that schooling was doing was trying to make me fit into society. All the testing they did was to find out what society wanted me to do, not what I wanted me to do. It was TLS that supported me in searching out a dream that I owned, not a cut-rate dream foisted off on me by some well-meaning case manager. It was TLS that offered the job courses and the job group and support center. It seems to have frequently been TLS that has been in the right place with the right support at the right time.

The most important thing you can do to get psychiatric patients working full-time is to find out what *they* want to do, not what various professionals think they ought to be doing. Don't tell us what we should be doing; ask us what we want to do.

At the Alliance, I work with other people like myself who have been in the mental health system. We share our common knowledge and experience to provide advocacy for other people in the system. We talk about choice, and options, and responsibilities. It is the best kind of peer advocacy: people who have been there, talking to people who are there. At the Alliance we work to eliminate the stigma of being a mental patient, and to treat each other with respect and dignity.

SIGNS*

Margaret Robison

I am not mad now.
But I remember the locked ward
and the women who would live their lives
and die there. I remember
screaming that went on and on
and wouldn't stop—
Sometimes it was the scream
of the woman with scars
from wrist to shoulder.
Sometimes it was the scream
of the woman behind the locked door
or the woman who wept for her cats.
Sometimes the scream was my own.

But I am not mad now.
And the crayon marks
on the ward ceiling
were after all
ancient signs
as I had known all along—circles,
squares, lines. Pure,
simple shapes in a childlike scrawl
and each of them said to me: *Live*.
Live.

---

* First appeared in *Slant*, Summer 1991 issue.

PART 3

STANDING OUR GROUND: THE POLITICAL CONTEXT OF "MADNESS"

If you are a psychiatric patient, it is assumed that there must be something seriously wrong with YOU. The psychiatric system would have us believe that there is no such thing as a political context of "madness": "Madness" happens in a vacuum; it results from biochemical or genetic abnormality; it has nothing to do with the rest of the world which is "normal" and immune—or so the story goes.

In a society that relies on scapegoats in order to function, this view of "madness" is very convenient. It assures the dominant power group's staying in power since it is they who decide what "normal" is in the first place. It also assures that the suffering will continue.

The writing in this section explores the political/social roots of "mental illness." Despite the popular belief that "madness" is biological in origin, the survivors in this section have a different story. From our experiences, "madness" has to do with homelessness, poverty, sexism, racism, ableism, mentalism, ageism, homophobia, ethnocentrism, and child abuse, to name a few.

The interaction among society, the mental health system, and the diagnosed "mentally ill" is complex. Much of it happens on the level of assumption and since the "mentally ill" are scapegoats par excellence, there is strong resistance to examining these assumptions. But invisible as the political context of "madness" may be to some, the facts are blatant; and the assumptions that lead to psychiatric oppression are detrimental to everyone.

The writers in this section show clearly that the politics of "madness" has EVERYTHING to do with "madness."

MONEY CHANGES EVERYTHING*

Dee dee Bloom

It took many months away from the misery entrepreneurs before I began to realize their effect on my life and on society as a whole. While paying a shrink, I drifted away from unpaid friends. I learned that not only did I frighten them, but that they lacked experience to help me understand my pain. I learned friends were "too close" to the situation, that I couldn't trust them with my deepest secrets. I learned that only thoughtless, self-centered people expect support for free from untrained folks they call friends. Friends learn from subtle behavior modification programming that turning to books, dogs, trees, streams, or deep breathing will only delay "necessary treatment" and worsen the potential customer's condition.

To believers, *therapy* means goodness, helpfulness, and expert care. No matter what goes wrong in the chatting-for-hire relationship, the opinions of the faithful do not budge. When one professional damages us, we often seek out another in hopes they'll fix us up and heal our pain from the previous damage. Torture, murder, brain washing, incarceration, rape, battering, and fascism all happen in the name of therapy. These are not merely side effects or the errors of misguided professionals. They are part of the package. All therapy is political and hierarchical. Some professionals lie about the relationship more than others.

---

* First appeared in *Sinister Wisdom 36*, Winter 1988/89 issue. This is an excerpt from *The Misery Business*, a book in progress.

Psychotherapy is a medicalized term used to distinguish it from common activities. If we play in our homes it's called play; if it occurs in a professional building, the identical activity becomes play therapy. If we weave baskets or make belts, we're doing art/craft labor; if under psychiatric guidance, we're engaging in occupational therapy. If we wash our kitchen floor, we're cleaning house; if we're inmates in a psychiatric institution, we're engaging in industrial therapy. The market is rapidly expanding to include every activity imaginable. People in this field can only make a living from what they perceive as therapy.

All universities teach beliefs. Beliefs become facts when the majority of those in power agree with the beliefs. The general population is often in awe of what it takes in time and resources to acquire a degree. People are taught to assume that a degreed person is better qualified, more skilled and dependable than her or his nondegreed counterpart. Less expensive and time-consuming ways exist to exchange ideas and teach each other different ways of doing things. But without social validation from degree-granting institutions, ordinary wisdom remains outside the realm of possibilities.

Universities do more than sell information. They create a professional privileged class and institutionalize racist, sexist, and classist ideologies. The concept of professionalism serves to divide the haves from the have-nots. To insist on the preface "doctor" for one's name is to desire the status of master over others. The ideologies of therapy and professionalism overlap in purpose and meaning. Both convey a sense of goodness and desirability. Hidden beneath this cloak of misinformation we find that both therapy and professionalism encourage inequality, authoritarianism (under the guise of expertise), cut-throat competition, and ethical irresponsibility. Simply by virtue of their titles alone professionals are considered respectable, trustworthy specialists. They teach lay people that oppression wears a smile and should be embraced and respected. They repeat the mantra to themselves and each other, "We are superior to nondegreed helpers and friends because of our expensive formal education. Everyone needs our services because all people have difficulties surviving in the modern world."

Why We Buy

New graduates of mental health industry training enter one of the fastest growing markets in advanced capitalism, thanks to government-sponsored advertising. We don't choose therapy simply because we're angry, hurt, frustrated, isolated, and confused. A manipulative and clearly planned advertising campaign financed by tax dollars continuously shapes our thinking on the subject. We learn almost hypnotically and unconsciously to associate the terms therapy, helpfulness, and alleviation of pain.

The media is the most powerful ally of the misery industry. Reporters present the beliefs and opinions of psychiatrists as scientific facts. Successes and breakthroughs are big news. Death and relapse make poor copy but are quite common.

Misery entrepreneurs use the media to their individual and collective advantage. Because they perceive that most problems have a personal solution that can be marketed as therapy, there is no end to supply and demand. Part of any advertising campaign is to make a product desirable and then to confuse a potential buyer about the difference between desire and need. The final step is to create a dependency on the product and limit its delivery to the marketplace.

Therapists require dependency from customers; they survive on it. Part of the professional's marketing strategy in collaboration with government agencies is to convince potential customers that, first, professional conversation is a service commodity and that, second, the populace desperately needs to buy what they alone are licensed to sell.

Language is another important aspect of the sale. Atrocities hidden in language are a method used by both the military and the mental illness industry to keep their image acceptable and saleable. Take for example psychiatric and psychological treatment. Many people think that when a person is placed in a locked facility with no trial, that inmate has been incarcerated illegally. If a medical staff runs the locked building, people believe, due to advertising, that the "patient requires hospitalization." Drugs are called "medication" when prescribed. Medications somehow avoid the current medical blitz on drug abuse. Supposedly only self-medicators abuse chemicals. Electrical shocks change to electroconvulsive therapy. When a person takes a razor and carves little lines into her arms, doctors call it self-mutilation. When a physician saws into a person's skull and slices out portions of the brain, doctors call it psychosurgery.

How many folks would bring their friends, their kin, or themselves to the prison gate for punishment? By medicalizing the language to "hospital," "treatment," and "help," authorities know that many will turn in themselves and their loved ones.

▲ ▲ ▲

In the office of the therapist, a more subtle form of oppression occurs. Equally dangerous, it too goes unrecognized and unchallenged. The expert promotes herself as different from and superior to the ordinary peer. Some therapists claim equality with their customers while promoting themselves as superior to the customer's peers. The medicalized title of the paid conversationalist or treater is central to the entire misery enterprise. Also important is the language professionals use to describe their customers. Some therapists call those who pay them *customers* or *clients*. These experts attempt to demedicalize the buyer's position in the hierarchy. Removing the stigma of *mental patient* is good for the business of those who fear the "real weirdos." They can treat everybody else. For some reason, these therapists see no reason to change their own title or position. They were top dog with patients and still are with client/customers. A change in title might have threatened their authority and therefore their income.

Psychotherapists today need the patronage of their customers and the State to survive economically in their career. Even though customers and the State keep them in the money, they pretend it is their product (therapy) that is needed. How many workers do you know who can charge for services their customers didn't order and don't even want, who can drag out the sale for a lifetime, and who control both the time and the manner in which their services are delivered to the market?

If a house cleaner who earns $10 an hour questions her psychotherapist who charges $85 for fifty minutes, the therapist may equate money with personal worth. "I charge $85 because I'm worth it. You would too if you could get it . . . and I can help you get what you want and deserve." More frequently, the discussion shifts to the customer's supposed problems. "Why do you resist my attempts to help you feel better? Why can't you make and keep commitments in your life?"

Once somebody lays their money on the table, the therapy hook goes deeper. Sellers congratulate their voluntary customers for "doing something good for yourself" or starting to "take care of yourself" and advise that "you owe this to yourself." The fee collector reminds customers that "this is a safe place, a nonjudgmental place. You need not censor a single verbal response." "You're not weird or alone." "It took great strength and courage for you to make the decision to come here today. I applaud your strength." "You're special. I'm here and I care." It's seductive to have an audience who you believe is there only for your well-being.

Therapists tell their customers to share their fears in this society, but in an attempt to mask their own terror, they drug visionary customers. Because most customers have learned to fear these nonordinary sensory perceptions, they willingly swallow damaging chemicals and hope the payoff is worth the risks. Drugs are well-marketed and highly profitable. Drugs prove how much users need them like therapists prove how much we all need therapy.

Government Dispensaries

Money is one of the most taboo topics in this commercial caring enterprise. Folks without money have "the right to treatment," but if professionals judge them or their middle-class counterparts as being possessed with a serious mind sickness, they have no right to refuse treatment.

Without choice, the legal system sends offenders to misery entrepreneurs as a court sentence, a requirement of parole, or an alternative to jail. Others go as a requirement for receiving public assistance, an insurance settlement, or so the court won't take away their children. As professionals have moved into the lucrative market of child psychiatry, more and more children are forced to participate in treatment. Over the past five years, child diagnoses have increased 1000% and child hospital admissions (incarcerations) have increased 400% over the same period.*

Social turmoil greatly benefits misery business entrepreneurs both in private practice and in clinics. The more who come to

---

* John McKnight, "A Nation of Clients," *Public Welfare*, fall 1980, pp. 15-19.

the clinics, the more clinics will be reimbursed by third-party payments. While the customer in private therapy for two years will pay ten times the amount of the annual income of half of humanity, the public customer also contributes to the gross national product. John McKnight writes that those receiving public assistance are more valuable in their dependency because so much income is derived from this dependency.* They probably will never produce the amount made off them, so cannot contribute as much working as they can dependent on services and therapy.

The government and the misery business need each other to survive. Misery entrepreneurs (including sellers who call themselves feminist and radical) adjust people to their oppression. In return, the government grants these professionals certain privileges, licenses, and free advertising. It is in their interest to conceptualize social injustice as individual psychopathology (mind sickness). It is in their interest to have the "masses" adjust to oppression. It is in their interests to train the "masses" to seek out authority for every problem and to make authority appear concerned with our well-being.

If we're all isolated and preoccupied with blaming ourselves for our poverty, homelessness, sickness, battering, and unhappiness, we will never unite and confront the unequal distribution of wealth, stealing disguised as taxation, biological warfare, racism, sexism, or anything else. We won't even recognize their existence. Social unrest and demands for equality will be put to rest in favor of a trip to the therapist. We all pay for such a philosophy. Some more than others.

Who's Sorry Now?

Sellers of therapy have a few formulas to deal with dissatisfied, violated, or dead customers. One is called "the bad apple" theory. They pull it out frequently because so much seems to go wrong in the misery business. The bad apple theory concedes that cruel or ignorant practitioners exist among professional ranks but that a few misguided and ill individuals

---

* John McKnight, "A Nation of Clients," *Public Welfare*, fall 1980, pp. 15-19.

in no way reflect on the entire operation, only happy endings and customer satisfaction.

Cooptation is an important aspect of diffusing anger and restraining social action against all institutions, including psychiatry and psychotherapy. Faithful customers diffuse criticism of the profession by accusing violated critics of poor shopping habits. "You just didn't find the right shrink." The assumption here is that there is choice at all times.

Entrepreneurs and customers also charge survivors of therapy violence with frightening the needy with horror stories, and they label critics as "mentally ill."

Feminists Strengthen the Business

Criticizing feminist conversation-for-hire in a meeting or a women's news journal in the United States is like criticizing Catholicism in the Vatican. Women jump to defend their shrink (feminist therapist) and shrinks jump to defend their products. The critic rapidly becomes viewed as the antifeminist, the outsider, the ignorant. Critics are too negative, unsupportive of women's needs, can't listen, and are "addicted" to an antitherapy stance—is the response of the pro-therapy community. If a feminist seller violates a customer, the feminist was only masquerading as a feminist or the incident never really happened. Unlike other sellers, feminists seem to believe that their colleagues never harm, disable, or destroy their customers.

The term *feminist* is not a liberating one to me. Further, I do not support the U.S. feminist therapy movement. A group so embedded in psychiatric jargon and one that takes no stand against incarceration is not a women's liberation movement. Maybe that's why they took "liberation" out of the name and decided to call themselves a feminist rather than a women's liberation movement. One friend of mine suggested that a change in class perspective put women's liberation out and feminist in as labels. I think the feminist therapy movement in the United States is different from women's liberation in other parts of the world.

Neither political criticism of psychiatry nor counterinstitutions were new ideas in the 1960s. Women's liberation theorists naively decided that the problem with psychiatric and psychological services was an overabundance of male practitioners treating female patients and a sexist theoretical foundation for such treatment.

With a limited analysis of the problem, no critique of a medicalized language, and little understanding of classism within the professions, women set up grassroots projects such as women's centers, battered women's shelters, and mutual support networks. They took power rather than waiting for the experts to "empower them" with the right to change.

Meanwhile, highly educated feminist entrepreneurs decided that the way to change the system and "empower" women was to work from within the system. This at least gave them a good salary compared to grassroots organizers who had to scramble for phone money. The reform philosophy is different from a philosophy of revolution. Their strategy was to reorganize existing institutions without altering their basic foundations. They called their reorganized institutions "alternatives." An alternative's progressive appearance helped appease certain elements of this social change movement.

Feminist therapy, for example, was conceptualized and marketed as an alternative to oppressive psychotherapy. All licensed sellers pay tuition in the same classist, racist, and sexist universities, but supposedly those calling themselves feminist put their indoctrination aside to bring their sisters a product packaged with more appeal. Feminist therapy sellers, in an effort to corner the market in the political women's community and convince prospective buyers of this therapy's uniqueness, proclaimed equality between buyers and sellers (some later acknowledged that it wasn't an equal relationship).

Is it equal when buyers teach sellers about human interactions and give them marketable experience yet have to pay to teach? Is it equal when buyers are expected to share their innermost secrets while sellers sit safely watching and interpreting their customers' behavior? If the seller decides to share pain and the buyer listens as part of her paid treatment? When one has the power to imprison the other?

Another early selling technique was to convince women with political problems that therapy could help. As a recruitment method, supporters of feminist therapy decided that political women could get politicized and active through feminist therapy, not through peer consciousness-raising groups or any other obviously political channel. Nondegreed women offering women feminist therapy for free needed to be dealt with. The pros taught trainees that working without economic remuneration was antifeminist and showed they suffered from a mother/martyr complex. Nondegreed women began charging women to come to groups in their homes, groups that in the past had been peer-organized without fees. Now professionals pointed out that they were selling support without a license and advised women to purchase proper university training.

Professionals were invited into many rape crisis centers and battered women's shelters to observe and help out as equals. Slowly they moved out the "lay persons" who organized the shelters in the beginning. Women wrote articles and sold workshops on how to choose a therapist. Professionals invented syndromes for survivors of rape, battering, and incest and wrote up grants to provide "treatments" for these diagnoses. They said that what women in pain, women battered and raped, women brutalized in prisons and psychiatric institutions need is not mutual support, grassroots organizing and political revolution. We need a marketable resource, an expert to chat with, a professional "sister" to sell us hope.

While inactively waiting for a revolution, frustrated feminists need to purchase professional talking. How else can one keep her spirits up in these unsettling times? Sellers make buying easy. A woman can even buy on a sliding scale from the majority of sellers, though they generally slide up easier than they slide down. Sliding scales are a great marketing strategy for a glutted market. Women who would otherwise pay nothing now pay something and feel gratitude for the favor.

In a relationship determined by money and inequality, women learn how to relate, to love, to befriend one another. Noncommercial relationships weaken as the therapeutic model of relating teaches women how to be (or not be) with each other. Feminist therapy sellers know that "the personal" makes better business sense than "the political." Classified sections in women's papers don't include "political growth" sections. The sellers market therapy as a social change activity. The government is pleased with the state of affairs. It supports the philosophy of capitalist individualism. This philosophy is based on the idea that personal change is really the only change possible and that social change as part of personal change is inconceivable. How can a hurting, confused woman even think about changing the social structure with others before she purchases and completes a lifelong personal care program?

Where Do We Go?

Those making war would definitely prefer to psychologize every aspect of our lives, for obvious reasons. If we're bombed it's because we have negative thoughts rather than greedy governments.

When we psychologize an inmate's anger or a critic's displeasure, we quit paying attention to these people. They become invisible. Psychotherapy has harmed many people and altered even our most intimate relationships. It helps all right: it helps us become more invisible to each other and to the government.

Disenchanted therapy customers often have difficulty finding each other, and psychiatrically violated people generally experience isolation, silence, and self-blame for atrocities not of our own making. This must and can stop. The solution is not to hire nondegreed therapists or hire peers to hear our pain. We can all start talking to each other outside the marketplace. Though it takes a lot of courage and attention, we can start changing the world today by asking a woman "how are you?" and meaning it.

Bibliography

Bergin, Allen E. "The Deterioration Effect: A Reply to Braucht," *Journal of Abnormal Psychology*, 75(3): 300-302. 1970.

Bergin, Allen E. "The Effects of Psychotherapy: Negative Results Revisited," *Journal of Counseling psychology*, 10(3): 244-250. 1963.

Cardea, Caryatis. "The Lesbian Revolution and the 50 Minute Hour: a Working Class Look at Therapy and the Movement," *Lesbian Ethics*, 1(3): 46-58. 1986.

Duxbury, Micky. "Feminist Therapy?" *Madness Network News*, 3(8): 16-17. 1975.

Evgenia, Tracie. "How Feminist Is Feminist Therapy?" *off our backs*, 6(6): 2-3+. 1976.

Feyerabend, Paul. "Experts in a Free Society," *The Critic*, Nov/Dec 1970, pp. 58-69.

Hadley, Suzanne W. and Strupp, Hans H. "Contemporary Views of Negative Effects in Psychotherapy," *Archives of General Psychiatry*, 33: 1291-1302. 1976.

Hoagland, Sarah Lucia. "Lesbian Ethics: Some Thoughts on Power in Our Interactions," *Lesbian Ethics,* 2(1): 4-32. 1986.

Hurvitz, Nathan. "Manifest and Latent Functions in Psychotherapy," *Journal of Consulting and Clinical Psychology,* 42(2): 301-302. 1974.

Hurvitz, Nathan. "Peer Self-Help Psychotherapy Groups and Their Implications for Psychotherapy," *Psychotherapy: Theory Research and Practice,* 7(1): 41-49. 1970.

Hurvitz, Nathan. "Psychotherapy as a Means of Social Control," *Journal of Consulting and Clinical Psychology,* 40(2): 332-339. 1974.

Kelly, Betsy. "Selling Yourself," *RT: a Journal of Radical Therapy,* 4(7): 10. 1975.

Lakoff, Robin Tolmach. "When Talk Is Not Cheap: Psychotherapy as Conversation," *The State of Language,* L. Michaels and C. Ricks (eds.), Berkeley: University of California Press, 1980, pp. 440-448.

Lee, Anna. "Therapy: the Evil Within," *Trivia: a Journal of Ideas,* 9: 34-45. 1986.

Lowenstein, Andrea Freud. "Kate Millet's Loony Bin Trip," *Sojourner,* June 1987, pp. 12-15.

Mancuso, J.C., et al. "Psychology in the Morals Marketplace: Role Dilemma for Community Psychologists," *A Consumer Approach to Community Psychology,* J.K. Morrison (ed.), Chicago: Nelson Hall, 1979, pp. 261-294.

Matarazzo, Joseph D. "Some Psychotherapists Make Patients Worse!" *International Journal of Psychiatry,* 3: 156-157. 1967.

McKnight, John. "A Nation of Clients," *Public Welfare,* Fall 1980, pp. 15-19.

Oden, Thomas. "A Populist's View of Psychotherapeutic Deprofessionalization," *Journal of Humanistic Psychology,* 14(2): 3-18. 1974.

Peck, M. Scott. *People of the Lie: The Hope for Healing Human Evil.* New York: Simon and Schuster, 1983.

Perenyi, Constance. "Enough Is Enough: Feminist Therapy and Other Bad Habits," *Big Mama Rag: a Feminist News Journal,* 7(1): 11, 20+. 1980.

Sullivan, Gail. "Women's Shelters House Contradictions," *Sojourner,* 7(8): 5. 1982.

SUICIDE: A VERB[*]

Catherine Odette

I feel great pressure to measure each word many times before I let it out and into this piece. I am frightened that the words will be too . . . oh, scary or maybe too . . . hmm, bold, or worse yet, too . . . damn, too small or just plain insufficient for the task of talking about suicide.

I worry that these words will carry a kind of contagion, an "ah, yes!" to someone who is in pain, whose remembering is a devastation, who has been waiting for an idea that will solve all her problems. I don't know how to protect us all from the contagion aspects of the discussion of suicide except to say clearly that I don't believe suicide is the solution to problems. So much of what our problems are is outside our control, is dumped on us to deal with—leaving us on the precarious edge between blaming ourselves for someone else's actions and feeling the guilt/shame/panic that is their legacy. The incest/family rapes, the sexual assaults, the homophobia, sexism, and more generally the misogyny that are given to all women but especially to lesbians; the racism, discrimination, sizeism, poverty; the barriers and direct methods created to destroy women's strength and encourage disempowerment . . . none of this is solved by our death.

These problems cannot be fixed by any single woman's death. Rather, each of these problems remains, but the person is no longer there to care about them or try to solve them. She

---

[*] First appeared in *Dykes, Disability and Stuff*, vol. 3, no. 1.

can no longer take an action to solve, fix, remedy, alter, change, eliminate, or eradicate the problem. She is no longer there to have the power that solving the thing might/will bring her.

This said, I move on to talk about suicide.

▲ ▲ ▲

I know a lot about wanting to suicide. You probably noticed right away that I didn't place the word *commit* in front of the word *suicide*. I think of the word *suicide* as a verb, a word that describes an action. I don't perceive suicide to be a criminal act. An unsuccessful suicide is an act very much like the acknowledged crime of "breaking and entering," which, when unsuccessful (that is, if you get caught), causes you punishment.

When you are, say, just a regular person, going about your own life, you have many rights. The right to (unsuccessfully) suicide is not among your rights. Suicide is a crime in every state of the United States. This crime can be and regularly is punished—if you are unsuccessful. Usually, if you are unsuccessful, you are considered sick—mentally sick—and you can generally expect to be hospitalized for a while in a place where all your human rights are abridged and/or suspended. Unless you can convince the powers-that-be that "it" was an accident or you can convince them of some other explanation for what they mistook to be suiciding, well, now you can count on spending time on a psychiatric unit of a general hospital or in a specifically "psychiatric" hospital.

If you are, say, a person with a disability, your right to suicide is mostly, quietly, nonverbally, nonspecifically, nondirectly, and nonlegally granted. Unless you need help doing it. Unless your disability is psychiatric. Unless someone else is your conservator (has the right to make your decisions for you). Unless you fail at suicide regularly. (You see why the words are so very important. I must say this "just so" the first time out.)

I have a powerful and terrifying relationship with suicide. I know so very much about how to do it. Many people in my life have chosen suicide. I have listened to them as they considered it. I have begged, cajoled, pleaded; I have acceded to their personal decisions both in favor of life and in favor of death. I believe in each person's right to choose suicide. I have terrible pain remembering my losses when others have exercised their right to suicide. I have been "rescued" from my own rightful effort to suicide.

I am glad to be here today talking about suicide, but I continue to rage against the circumstance that I was left with—because I was unsuccessful. It took me years to be really glad to have lived. Beth D. says she is always "recovering from suicide," because every day's struggle with the ideas and feelings of suicide exact immense pain, energy, and work.

The wish to suicide is fodder for many potent tearjerker movies about people with disabilities. The story about the paint artist who is now quadriplegic—and who can't imagine life without being able to paint—petitions the court: "How would you like it if you had to be me?" pleads the character. The rap of the gavel stops the forced feedings or the involuntary medication or respirator or whatever life support treatments are going on. The viewing public breathes for the first time in almost 90 minutes (excluding commercials) as approval for a disabled person to "disappear" is meted out. "Life with disability is not worth living" is the message. "There is no way for a disabled person to be an artist" is another message. The judge is clear: "If you were a real (whole) person, I would wonder at your sanity, I would think you crazy, but since you aren't real (whole) and since life with a disability IS worthless, you are not only not crazy, but (YOU) are within your rights to die. The state grants you the right to find a way to suicide."

"Now, if you WERE crazy," says some fictitious judge, "and we are clear that I, a judge and probably a stranger, get to say whether you're crazy, then we, the legal and the psychiatric systems, would work really hard and almost certainly prevent you—at any cost—from killing yourself. We have special hospitals, with rooms designed to keep you from hurting yourself. We have mind-altering drugs, brain-damaging shock treatments, unskilled, often brutal attendant/guards who will zealously keep you from killing yourself . . . even if that should take us the rest of your life." In a bizarre twist, in that marriage of ableism and mentalism, the same argument to keep you from dying when and how you might choose will force you into the horrific abuse of a "mental" institution, possibly for the rest of your life.

I am reminded of who my peers would be in a court of (men's) law. It would not be twelve (good and true) separatist dykes with varying disabilities. Nooooo indeed. It would not be twelve strong lesbian disability allies. It would not even be twelve women, because every woman knows too much about

sexual abuse, about misogyny, about living outside herself and
trying to diet, bend, squeeze, and paint her way to acceptance
in this woman-hating world. When I think about who may
"judge" my actions, I finally, fully, absurdly comprehend
patriarchy.

▲ ▲ ▲

I live with suicide. I know people today who may choose
suicide any minute. I perceive their decisions as deeply rational,
deeply thought out, and deeply personal. They talk about
suiciding as a defense and solution to their pain. They
understand that the things causing the pain will not be
eliminated. They understand that suiciding means that *they* will
be eliminated. Mostly, their lives are not horrible (they tell me).
Mostly, this is a choice they describe as "the ultimate control"
or "being in charge" of their lives. I understand in a most
personal way about this control stuff and this being in charge
stuff.

OK. Here it is. The part I didn't want to talk about. I have
both physical disabilities and psychiatric disability. I have no
problem saying those things. I have no shame over any of my
disability stuff. I even feel glad about being a person with
disabilities (though not about the inhumane
institutionalizations). I am unique in who I am because of the
stuff of my life. I feel like an authority on some things, having
lived such extremes of them in my lifetime. But the quality of
my life is always being defined by someone ELSE! If I were the
one to choose what is working for me and/or what is successful,
I would always have options and choices. So often, my world
has impossible barriers and useless nonchoices. It's not that just
a bit of elbow grease or a scintilla more push or more thought
or more something or a bigger something else or better some
other thing would fix things. Sometimes it's all just beyond me.

So, sometimes, yes indeed, often, the idea of suicide has its
attraction. I would have to be really splashy about it, I think.
Nowadays, it's my style to make every moment count double,
triple, quadruple, or more. I don't exactly know what I mean,
but I'm sure every pocket of my clothing would be filled with
notes, proofs, and damning letters to parties guilty of some of
the world's ills. I reserve the right to NEVER be at the mercy of
life's institutions again.

▲ ▲ ▲

I treasure my right to suicide. I am ill at the pain that one's suicide leaves for others.

It is so hard to say good-bye. Someone who dies is really gone forever. I can't stand that sometimes. When I want to talk to Susan or Rita, their not being here is so painful. I still feel their deaths. I unwillingly imagine their last moment, that final exhalation, and I want to push it back into them, to have them somehow make really sure one more time before they suicide and leave me behind. What can I possibly do or say or think that makes being left behind less painful? After all these years, news of another dyke's suicide still tears at that unhealed chamber of my heart, the one reserved for saying good-bye, that place where understanding and regret have both made a home.

Learning about a dyke's death is terrible, even if all I know about her is that she was a dyke. The death of a dyke forces us to celebrate her life without her. It's really hard to do it well. Learning about a dyke's suicide will always leave me teary. I put a whisper on the wind for her, sending a breath of understanding for the choice, for the exercising of a right that would have been stolen from her, if she had lived.

I still feel great pressure to measure each word many times before I let it out. I am frightened that my words will be too . . . oh, scary or maybe too . . . hmm, bold or worse yet, too . . . too damn small and insufficient for the task of talking about suicide.

OCTOBER POEM

(on my birthday)

Jodi Lundgren

I'm scared and I want
to write poetry
on the back of bills and receipts
to eat chocolates
under a quilt
till I'm too fat to fit through the door.
I want to screen all my calls
hide behind my bear
and read only books that don't remind me
of my life.
I want to wear two thick sweaters
as shields against the pain.
I want to smother the clock with blankets
to silence its ticking.
I want to spin myself a wool cocoon
then hibernate through the dark time,
dreaming long avenues of trees
where sun illumines
bright yellow leaves.

I want to stop stepping on nails
and gouging stigmata into my feet.
I never said I was the reincarnation
of Jesus—that was your misconception.

I don't want to make up stories
to talk around the truth.

Now it's time to strip away denial.
I've learned to read
my chronic sore throats
as symptoms, not as sickness.
I couldn't stop them
when I was six
they cut my tonsils out.
But now I have the power to resist.
It's not the way you saw it
with your Pollyanna view.
You taught us to delete the sordid
from tales we brought you at table
like dead mice on a doormat,
and I knew better than to ask the meanings of words.
I read the newspaper, used a dictionary,
and thought rape had just been invented
when I discovered what it meant.

Even now sleep pushes dreamy folds at me,
wanting to suck me under.
My psyche says, don't tire me,
don't push me, probe me, press me,
don't search for the truth—there isn't one.
Everyone remembers differently.

I need encouragement, sage advice,
from someone who enters the dark
and keeps on pushing

as jerking shaking milkshake making mouth wide open
for the dentist eyes closed lids red throat jammed
rough scratchy hair drowning going to die this time
bitter taste down my throat washed away with red
    Koolaid
my favorite.

Squished under my father's desk—
that space I could almost stand in—
in the den before my sister was born and my brother took
    over
the room, barred from me on pain of death.
A polished wood-chip on a leather thong

hung on his bulletin board, printed "MASTER"
in calligraphic script. I flipped it over to read "SLAVE."
The dyad gripped the pit of my belly.
That room.
That orange bucket chair.

Tinkerbell lived inside the chandelier—
"Leave the hall light on"—
that hung, inaccessible, over the stairwell.
I could just see the smoked glass, a protected world,
    through the crack in my door.
If I called her,
she'd come running down the hall
in her nightgown to save me.
When I finally tested my theory,
I yelled, "Mom! Mom!"
Always a light sleeper
she was deaf to my voice.

My sister and I tried to control our "illnesses"
we knew "doctor" meant "idiot."
Anorexia,
manic-depression
labels we shucked and fought.

We knew what the problem was.
We wanted to control what we couldn't before.
Take our lives into our own hands.
But no one's words addressed us.
We weren't seen or heard.
As children, we always wanted
to hide inside forts and tents,
or climb high into leafy trees.
Be safe.

Dad, you thought nothing mattered
that happened to a child;
she wouldn't remember when she grew up.
Then, she'd only be grateful, she'd only be good,
bring you home As on report cards
and success in the world
(dead birds on a doormat).

Well, I don't want to suck your dick;
your perversion isn't mine.
Even when I told you this,
falling on my knees,
you found a way to blame me.
You struck my head from side to side
till I passed out and both of you
walked out of my life.

I was the one who was locked up;
I was the one who was drugged.
You visited me in the hospital,
but disclaimed responsibility,
didn't understand my state of mind.
The male doctor prescribed antipsychotics
(the problem was chemical)
and handed the paper to you, Dad, the chemist.
I was sealed inside the system
slipped slyly back and forth
while everyone kept "Mum"
and turned their faces the other way.
The medical authorities complied with
YOU, the rapist
of your own child.

Listen to me, Dad,
I won't let you put this down.
I'm going to scream this from the rooftops
of a safe feminist stronghold.
I shot you in my dream last night,
repeatedly, deliberately.
You betrayed me!
Assaulted me, then turned me in
let them pump me full of drugs.
No one listened
as the word "incest" passed my lips.
Oh, you heard me, Dad,
but hushed me with your "No."
As though I would forget it all,
as though your magic tranquilizers
would plunge me into a fog

and silence me for the rest of my life.
You thought to sacrifice me
with impunity, like Iphigenia
but you forgot Philomela:
her tongue cut out, she wove the truth
of her rape
in brightly colored threads.

I came to the river today
hoping for movement and fresh breezes,
but the gray blanket of cloud
has sealed me in with pollution and humidity.
Even the river inches sluggishly.
Sometimes the oppression
is inescapable.
It unfolds from inside me, masking all.
I search for the source of this mess
and a place to release it.
Now I know the locus is YOU.
I protected you and Mom,
kept the family secret,
so we could be a Brady bunch—
two boys and two girls
with hair of gold
hearts of stone.

I won't carry the shadow any longer.
You remember, "the truth will out."
Out, out, damned spot!
I refuse the blemish.
I am rubbing off the tarnish
left by the abuse.
And you should see me shine, sir,
brighter than a new-minted coin
I'm shining like the dawn sun
that rose on the day I was born.
I'm glowing like the harvest moon
that set on that same night.

ELECTROSHOCK

A Modern Medical Atrocity*

Janet Gotkin

Between 1961 and 1971, I had more than 100 shock treatments, some with anesthesia, some without, in public hospitals and private institutions. I never signed a consent form and was never told what the procedure would consist of or what lasting debilitating effects I might endure.

In some ways I am rather a miraculous case. I survived more than 100 electrical assaults on my brain. Oh yes, I have large, unpredictable blank spots in my life history, unexpected, gaping, empty spaces I cannot fill. But years of drugs and shock did *not* destroy my body or my brain, did not incapacitate me as they have so many thousands of others.

Yes, ECT caused me excruciating pain, both psychic and physical, but I *did* emerge intact. I was very lucky. And I have felt, by virtue of this dumb luck—or perhaps sheer physical resilience—that I owe it to my less lucky sisters and brothers to

---

* This talk, by and large in this form, was presented at the First International Conference on Electroconvulsive Therapy (ECT): Clinical and Basic Research Issues, sponsored by the New York Academy of Sciences and the National Institute of Mental Health in New York City on January 16-18, 1985. Not a single opponent or questioner or survivor of electroshock had been invited to appear at the conference, but strenuous efforts by Bill Cliadakis and others resulted in conference organizers granting a "survivors' panel" one hour during the lunch break on the last day.

speak out on their behalf. In a sense, to tell their stories. All of our stories.

I've asked myself these things many times—and never successfully answered—questions about the people who give ECT, the "shock doctors": "Are these men evil?" I asked, using "men" since 95 percent of all shock doctors are male. "Are they stupid? Are they really heartless and sadistic and cruel? Are they morally deficient? Or, perhaps, do they suffer from a kind of self-induced blindness, and unwillingness to see what they are truly doing to the people they purport to help?"

I have always been unable to answer these questions fully and to the extent that I did, the answers did not shed any light on the phenomenon of men devoted to a profession of healing who embark upon and continue to practice a procedure that causes the kind of wholesale suffering and damage of ECT. Finally, I choose to be charitable and, rather than assuming malicious intent, assume a kind of benign but powerful avoidance on the part of these shock doctors of some painful truths about the nature of their chosen "therapy." We must tell some of those truths, in the belief that all people are capable of change, that all people can, if they truly want, be open to new ideas and long hidden truths.

As I tell my story, and others tell theirs, you can easily dismiss us with that once picturesque and now pejorative phrase that says our accounts are "anecdotal" and therefore meaningless. We, in turn, can counter by saying that the "clinical impressions" that doctors use to assess our "progress" are also anecdotal—and both sides can, in effect, cancel each other out.

Instead, I urge you to listen to what I have to say—and be aware that my testimony, my story, is only one of thousands—and that I speak, rather than someone else, because and only because I am a lucky, articulate, and favored survivor—for those who cannot or are afraid to speak for themselves.

▲ ▲ ▲

Each year, by their own estimate, ECT doctors shock at least 100,000 people. Seventy percent of those shocked are women and, by conservative estimates, 80 to 85 percent of them are over 65. At least 70 percent of them are fully covered by medical insurance. If we figure, again conservatively, that each of these people will receive ten to twelve shocks and will spend three to four weeks in a hospital, we can safely estimate that each of the 100,000 individuals will incur a bill of at least $10,000. In other words, each year, the practice of ECT and its concomitant hospitalization yields ONE BILLION DOLLARS.

After I did this figuring I was staggered, quite literally, by the sum. In spite of knowing that ECT doctors earn an average of twice that of general psychiatrists, I was, if you'll forgive me, shocked. That is an awful lot of money. It made me think—and question. Who are these 100,000? What are they paying for? What are they receiving?

You may not want to hear what I am going to say. You may wish to again indulge in self-induced selective deafness. But I will tell you who receives ECT: the most vulnerable and helpless people in our society. The most passive, the least likely to resist. The feeble, the old, the lonely, the disspirited. You may counter by saying that women and elderly people suffer more frequently from depression and thus are likely candidates for shock. But I tell you that we know better. We know better.

We have been coerced, we have been misinformed, we have been labeled and forced or maneuvered into undergoing your procedures, euphemistically called "treatments." Some of us, like me, have resumed our lives, emerging relatively unscathed. Very many others have not.

Yes, ECT "treatment" is a lucrative one, and ECT doctors congratulate themselves on the humanitarian and noble impulses that motivate their giving ECT. They discount our stories of loss. They turn deaf ears to inchoate pleas to stop. And they continue to try to give scientific credence to a procedure whose efficacy, after more than 35 years, is still completely undemonstrated.

What has been "proved"? I will tell you: that ECT destroys healthy brain tissue! That these "treatments" cause anguish and misery and permanent damage each and every time they are inflicted. That there are no consistent criteria for improvement, that patient accounts of memory loss and suffering are discounted—for elderly people, as signs of senility; for the rest of us, as indications that our so-called mental illnesses remain, unabated.

Who gets "well" from ECT? I will tell you: those whose confusion is so intense they can, for a while, forget their sufferings. Those who are incapacitated into a passive acceptance of their allotted roles. Those who are cowed into quietness, assaulted into a nether world of obedience. For a time, their wild, mad, annoying rambunctiousness is quelled—and the doctors marvel at their "improvement."

They bloody us into quietude, terrorize us into acquiescence, and call it a cure.

For sure, the ECT doctors are engaged in a highly questionable activity, both medically and ethically. And a profoundly controversial one. There really is no getting away from that. They can hold self-congratulatory conferences and not include anyone but their most ardent supporters, but the questions and issues do not go away! Do they tell their patients, ever, the price of the trade-off—permanent brain damage for possible temporary relief from pain? Do they say that they are systematically and methodically burning portions of their patients' brains—for a possible moment's surcease? *Do they tell themselves? Ever?*

A WOMAN ON SOCIETY'S TERMS

I Was Once an Independent Female, Now I Am a Tamed Shrew[*]

Batya Weinbaum

Inductive reasoning is when you go from the particulars of the experience to the general principle. From the small to the large. From the incident to the rule. From the inside out.

This essay is about the impact of institutionalization, or how the mental hospital experience, supposedly designed to make people better, makes many worse.

I am qualified to write this paper for several reasons. I have been in therapy, various kinds, off and on for five years, the past year and a half of which included four institutionalizations in a community mental health center under what the psychiatric profession would deem optimal conditions—family near, plenty of personal visits, and the attention of a genuinely concerned psychiatrist. All through the experience I read books—*The Politics of Experience* by R.D. Laing; the various popular novels about the experience by Gordon, for example, and Marge Piercy; Bateson's *Ecology of Mind*; books on depression; psychiatric books delineating the "borderline" symptoms. Finally, over the past six months I began to read sociological studies about mental institutions. I am still trying to understand *why* (the madman's question, as defined by the culture; see *Zen*

[*] First appeared in *Big Mama Rag*, May 1982.

197

and the Art of Motorcycle Maintenance) I got involved in the institutionalization process and why I am so scarred by it.

My qualifications for generalizing to theoretical explanations based on this personal experience also stem from the fact that I have had a lot of experience theorizing. From the fact, I say. Not from delusions of grandeur, not from exaggeration or distortion—but from the genuine factual reality that I am a widely published feminist theorist. When I generalize from my experience, or reason inductively to explain the social reality I live through in a new way, people buy what I have to say. They read it. They pay me money to come and speak to them, to explain to them even further the dynamics of how I think the system—particularly around production and reproduction of sex roles—works. In fact once, when in the hospital, I got an invitation to keynote a conference about women in the Netherlands: talk about juxtaposition of opposites, perceiving things in the extreme, black and white, high and low. In short, when I come up with interpretations, other people tend to agree with me and speak about how I make their experience of the world, if not more bearable, at least more meaningful.

I emphasize this fact for those who will discount what I will say because I was stupid enough to play the mental patient in life's theatrics of the absurd. That makes what I have to say irrelevant and unbelievable, you or society tell me. What I have to say is automatically discarded and swept away, read or interpreted or heard as yet another manifestation of another symptom. In fact, at times, even I have been convinced that for several years the theories I was making up were nothing more than my schizophrenic ideas of reference. Once in lockup, (euphemistically called "special care" on the unit) a guard (euphemistically redesignated "psych tech") said to me point blank that there was no such thing as feminist theory. He was sane, functioning; I was not; that I believed in my work was an incidence of my own insanity, he thought; in vain I disagreed with him.

That was *before* the wearing down of the hospital had really gotten to me.

▲ ▲ ▲

What kind of feedback did I get in the hospital that reduced me to believing an uninformed psych tech's word? A chorus of

mixed voices from patients, friends, family, staff, and doctor:
put away my writing, stop writing books, give up all this
liberated woman bullshit; what I needed was a man, somebody
else to anchor me, to have children; wear makeup, go the beauty
parlor, wear my hair in curls; go into the helping professions,
love my mother, learn to communicate with my family; channel
myself in a new direction, stop taking initiative, be passive,
dependent, and obedient; stop thinking, stop being intellectual,
put love before work, personal relations before need for shelter,
other people before self, emotional needs before career
ambitions; put off graduate school, do things for other people,
get into daily activities provided for me, cooking; stop making
decisions, let other people take care of me. I was no authority,
others knew more than I what was best for me.

In short what I got was a cancellation of myself, or the parts
of me that my adult self had struggled to be, and encouragement
to become the culture's definition of womanhood and
femininity, synonymous with being a mental patient, or so it
appears to me.

Consider the classic stereotype: can't make decisions, gets
identity through other people; economically irresponsible; prone
to emotional outbursts; gets off the topic easily; can't be
coherent or logical; gets distracted easily; opinion of self based
on opinion held by other people; ignorant of how the world
works; oversensitive; cries easily; given to hysteria.

But is that the stereotype of the female, or the mental
patient? It seems the same to me.

Because trying to shove me into the stereotypic female role
was such a rough fit, I became at once both. I once was an
independent female; now I am a tamed shrew. That's the
"humanizing" effect the hospital had on me.

But the independent female—let's evaluate just how far I was
in before this nervous breakdown or more politely called
"depression" hit me after the publication of my first book.[*]
What I experienced after the book came out was more or less a
loss of gender identity. Back in New York where I had been living
and where my problems began, I was used to having my life

---

[*] *The Curious Courtship of Women's Liberation and Socialism* (Boston:
South End Press, 1978).

center around intellectual relations with women. I was too self-directed, smart, and ambitious for many men. For example, I protested when parking my car that a date would grab the steering wheel and turn it right in my hands, explaining he was "just trying to help me" innocently. Or when someone else would want to decide what I should eat for me, or offer me his coat needlessly. Or when I would say I felt comfortable wearing a scarf, and a date would whip it off of my head, the better to look at me.

These are all small items, but they indicate my low tolerance for the "typical" male behaviors. They tend to want to take care of you and turn you into a decorative item that exists for them. Once I asked a man if he wanted to have children. Yes, he answered abashed, how did I know, he wondered, admiring my perceptive qualities. "Because you are treating me like one," I answered him. Needless to say, that relationship didn't last.

Before entering the hospital, I was typing up my journal, largely filled with anecdotes about my search for a man, and calling it *Notes on Psychotic Men by a Psychotic Woman: Or Dating in New York*. Somehow with the publication of my book, the intensity of my search became worse.

This worsening was partly a response to society's confusion about how to react to a woman's coming-out-as-an-intellectual ritual. The reaction of society's primary indoctrinating unit, the family, was typical. My parents reacted to this plateau in my career by wanting to take care of me. My mother was insulted and offended (as she usually is by me) that I was able to organize my book party by myself. After all, her services had been necessary to organize my brother's wedding for him, completely. My father started to give me money and wanted to buy me a coat—his symbol of wanting to protect me. I was made to feel guilty, rejecting his economic offers of assistance at first, as if I were crazy for wanting to do things on my own and in my own way. My brother and his wife, though invited, did not come to my book party, and when I asked my father why not, my father informed me, "Don't worry, they'll come to your wedding." Although I hadn't planned one.

Given my success as a writer but my failure as a woman on society's terms, this made me feel worse. At the book party, I was told I looked like a bride, as if wearing something borrowed, something old, something new and something blue. I invited every man I had gone out with throughout my seven years in

New York, frantically covering for the lack of a single partner. The shrink I was seeing came pregnant to the party, at which I served vodka and knishes, a Jewish dish frequently served at rituals. Her pregnancy with a child seemed to diminish the importance of the birth of my book.

I began to fly around the country to do speaking engagements, and when going through the Midwest, stopped to visit my parents. When was I going to have a baby, my mother's cleaning lady asked me; flippant then, I asked, when was she going to write a book. But each time I flew back to my loft in New York, I longed for a baby, a man, and resolutely pursued the building of my career based on my accomplishments, wondering if it really had been my success which was putting them off.

I was dumb, hopeful, and ambitious—then. I thought that I had constructed a step in my career, and I proceeded to try to build on it. But no. This is what led to my breakdown or depression, what I call the gap between consciousness and social identity. This gap creates the craziness in this world, and in extreme cases such as mine produces the mental patient.

In my consciousness, Book One should have led to Book Two, and the rewards should have been greater, not less. Doors should have opened for me as a result of my own success, not dictated by the mores of medieval chivalry. Instead I was unable to market the ideas for my second book successfully and was backed into doing a series of odd jobs once again. And except for a few women's publications, I could not get Book One reviewed.

Instead of building up, I had fallen down. My consciousness might have been using the sports metaphor of building up, rung to rung, add another ten pushups every workout, but since the ladder of patriarchal social hierarchy does not include a foothold for women's work, domestic or public, instead of stepping up, I had fallen down.

And I had fallen flat. The cost of living went up, while my capacity to earn went down in spite of my accomplishments. Was this what success had brought me? I had the same feeling as I did when as a child I tried to crawl upstairs to the second floor of my parents' two-story house. My brother, the elder by three years and always violent to me, threw me back down just as I reached the top of the stairs. I experienced terror, reeling backward. When I hit the bottom, my mother didn't pick me up or touch me, but towering above, hands on hips, asked, "Whose fault is this? Come on! Stop crying! Tell me! I've had enough of this!"

But there was no mother at the bottom now. No one to hit up against, not like when as a child in frustration I hit my head against the wall. The only one to hit up against was myself.

Following thoughts, which used to be a liberating process learned in therapy from my first shrink, became dangerous for me. Following thoughts in my mind became like restless wandering in a dangerous city. One wrong turn, and I'd be in a bad neighborhood. My mind, which had once been like an octopus with eight eyes wandering, became a blank.

I became afraid to go on the streets. I began to pick up men just to maneuver around, to get home from work or just to get from post office to store on one of my jobs. I decided to get out of New York. I used the money my father had given me to go to an artists' colony to try to re-center myself by writing, as writing was a way I had gained control and mastery in my life previously.

Little did I know my problems would follow me. I became afraid to drive. I found I couldn't control the ups and downs, the free associating in the car. I was trying to finish a second book, a theory of the workplace largely developed by firsthand observations and analysis of personal experience. I continued to develop the paradigm I was writing about, analyzing my current New York jobs, or the ones I was leaving; and I was writing about the process of theory development—my own—as well. But I began to have the feeling that I was being driven to the back of my mind by the women's movement. Not only was I conscious of the personal basis of the theory (which is more than most men are) but I was exposing myself by writing about it. Luckily I knew people would be interested in my story. Even so, the intensity with which I was writing and struggling with my own confusion and passion was evident to all around me.

My parents began to tell me to come home (a small town in the Midwest, home to them and where my childhood had been) to go to the hospital. I was scared, so it sounded good, but I knew it was wrong. My mother described the hospital (she worked for a branch of it) as a simple place where you withdrew to reevaluate goals. That sounded nice, safe; I had left the shrink I was seeing in New York. When you are seeing people who you are not sure are there and hearing them talk to you on the subways, no one understands you. Not even the therapist who had been supportive and understanding for so many years. She said I was hallucinating just to try to get her to mother me, that I was competing with her baby by my colossal disfunctioning.

That's all well and theoretically nice, but when you are getting lost in the streets, it doesn't help you. At this point I began to realize that there is violence involved in the so-called therapeutic relation. As with Marxism, an intellectual trend I had held much interest in, there is violence involved in the purest execution of the theory, and not everyone can deal with violence. If workers were to take over the factories as Marxism suggests, half of them would get shot. Workers know this, so they don't do it. Therapy patients are more vulnerable. They get hooked on completely trusting basically irresponsible individuals who eventually—no matter what the brand of therapy—misuse that trust. The therapists do this in two ways: by accusing you of an unwarranted dependency, which they have encouraged in you; or by asking you where you have gotten the unrealistic illusions they have implanted in you.

When I left my therapist in New York, I turned to friends, and this put great stress on my relationships. I knew this and I felt like I was losing people from my unnatural need to cling to them to batten down my own hysteria and to constantly go over decisions with them. My father's voice tempted me on the phone. "Come home and see Dr. **; he'll come right to the house to see you." You know it's wrong to let fathers take care of you, but you are scared—of going out, of breaking down to total strangers. You get there, and the doctor reassures you—that's what fathers are for. "It's all right to want to be cared for. Maybe you need it."

Before I tried to enter a hospital in New York on my own for the first time in the middle of all this, I had grabbed two of my topical notebooks (I kept running notebooks on different themes at the time). Audience and Femininity. I was extremely conscious of my use of flirtation as a connection to other people during this whole time. The immediate contact kept my mind from spinning. Instead of writing about sex roles for the far-away audience of the book, I was compulsively acting them out for whomever would look. I was quite conscious of the sexual connection to the psychiatrist in the hospital serving the same function for me. Here was a man who would be my audience, and listen to me. He was offering to take me in like

the hero in a Victorian novel. He was taking responsibility for
me. Here was a man who accepted my flightiness, confusion,
my femininity—and even seemed amused at it in me. I made a
lump transfer of trust to him, although I was uncomfortable
having done that and fought it constantly.

In *I'm Dancing As Fast As I Can*, Barbara Gordon has
written about how women are more likely to fall victim to the
psychiatric professional ritual. In my case, becoming a classic
female and a mental patient coincided pretty exactly. I became
a mental patient so to speak, to get my female gender identity
back, since publishing an intellectual book had pretty much
shaken it for me. I got into an intense relationship with a male
psychiatrist because I didn't like what my feminist consciousness
told me. With his help, I tried to batten it back down. Relating
to this male consistently paying attention to me gave me hope
that I too could be a success as a female.

Given the severity of sexism among men, the male
psychiatrist becomes a utopian alternative, especially attractive
to the woman who is out of her traditional gender role and thus
experiencing identity confusion. He is kind, and assures me,
trying to say with his patience and presence that all men are not
out to screw me. This was, in my case, in stark opposition to
my own raw experience in unmediated, impure life, and with
the rest of the men on the unit who began to hassle me as soon
as I was checked in on the first night. The first night, comments
were made about my appearance, which I was hostile to, and I
was accused of being a lesbian. Juxtaposed to that was the kind,
fatherly, protective type, and I felt relieved to be accepted and
understood by him. I stayed, responding to his pleas that I
needed him and exclaimed that I would rather die than go to
Massachusetts to return to my work, or to a university that was
offering me a low-paying fellowship to continue being a female
intellectual. He stepped into my patriarchally-induced
ambivalence about accepting my own individual overturning of
the gender role. I walked into the trap of which he was an
unknown enactor. I rejected my own work, choosing instead a
passive dependence on him, the savior, the psychiatrist.

THE HYPNOTIST

Batya Weinbaum

That's the world lady
you gotta lie if you wanna live in it.

She considered this good advice.

She went to the hypnotist.
You can hypnotize to change habits? she asked.

Yes, he answered.
I can hypnotize to not feel the pain
when I drive this nail into my hand—thus!

Listlessly she watched the blood squirm from him.

Good, she said.
I want to be hypnotized to act differently than my feelings.

Why no, he answered
to change your feelings you have to change what you
    think.

No, she answered,
I know what I think
and what I think is fine.
Men have been trying to change what I think for years.
I know what I feel and I have to learn to act differently.

She enunciated the words quite clearly.

Why, he answered,
diving into his black bag
to pull out his red satin
cloaking himself
in his own fantasy
of male omnipotence,
Others have tried, but I—

All men have to offer is sports metaphors and illusions,
    she insisted,
and I want none of them.

But I belong to all these organizations, he faltered.
I can change your thinking—
that's what's best for you.

I believe I know what's best,
she became belligerent.

That's like a patient saying, Doctor! Perform this
    operation on me!

Some people believe in patients' rights, she said.

I want to be hypnotized to say I can when I say I can't
to walk tall and proud and at a clipped pace down the
    streets
to not act as if I were invisible
just because others don't see or hear me.
I'll write the programs
you do the tricks
that's all I ask.

Go elsewhere young lady.

It's your world, she answered
I'm just trying to live in it.
He put away cape and gloves.

She went away doomed to a life of a stillborn white rabbit.

THE "E" WORD*

Rae E. Unzicker

This is a true story.

I was attending a mental health conference somewhere and happened on a workshop about "empowerment." Because the presenter was a mental health professional (a Ph.D. psychologist) practicing in a state hospital, who also called himself a "mental health consumer" (schizophrenic), I was interested in how he might address the inherent conflict of interest in the ideology of "empowerment." He told a story I found apocryphal, a story of how he "empowered" a client by "convincing" her to take her drugs, drugs that she clearly didn't want, that she had flatly refused, and that had caused her serious debilitating side effects. This was his idea of "empowerment."

Empowerment is a term bandied about by just about everybody in the disability movement, and it's been picked up in the "real world" and used as a weapon against oppressed people. For example, some conservative politicians want to remove single mothers from the welfare rolls, thereby "empowering" them to make it on their own. In any other country, this would be called slavery: in the new U.S. lexicon, it is called empowerment. The word has been trivialized into meaninglessness.

Professional advocates talk about empowering their clients when they're actually, at best, acting on behalf of their clients' expressed interests and, at worst, making decisions of their own

---

* First appeared in *The Rights Tenet*, Autumn 1993.

on behalf of a client whom they feel is not capable of making "responsible" decisions. Professionals also like to "empower" clients by giving them ersatz responsibility. A New York advocate boasts that, "One group is running the rehabilitation program every Sunday for a psychiatric center." One wonders if this is promoted in the name of empowerment or whether the center simply couldn't convince its professional workers to work on Sunday. One wonders whether the group is being paid to do the work at the same rate mental health professionals might be paid, with overtime for weekend work. One wonders why this group, if it is so "empowered," would accede to this tokenism when it clearly has no authority to hire and fire the regular staff.

Empowerment is a tricky word to begin with, because it is not a thing that can be given to another individual, like a gift or a piece of wisdom. Nor is it something one person can do for another. Empowerment is a totally personal process, one that evolves from the inside out. It is frequently motivated by personal outrage over intolerable conditions and, for a while, is expressed as anger. A lot of this occurred in the beginning of the mental patients' rights movement, and I believe that anger is still a primary and positive motivating force for change.

True empowerment rises up on its own out of pain, rage, and, most importantly, the individual's ultimate ownership of his or her own experience. Empowerment liberates. Empowerment facilitates recovery, not "acceptance of one's illness." Empowerment strengthens the voice, fortifies the will, and underscores hope. Empowerment is life-affirming. Empowerment is satori—that "aha!" in which one's personal truth is validated and honored from within. Empowerment thrives in an environment of freedom, integrity, and honesty. Empowerment does not occur in mental health facilities. True empowerment usually occurs, in fact, as a direct result of consciousness-raising, which almost always leads to the acknowledgement of and resistance to oppression.

Some people say that language is nothing, but language is everything. Perhaps, given a changing political climate, we can open a window in time and reclaim the word *empowerment*, with all it implies, for ourselves.

A REFUGEE IN
MY OWN COUNTRY

Janice L. Norman

I
have a voice.
It is part
of a national voice.
I have problems
you cannot see.
You can see my clothes
and stiff behavior.
When you see this
I see you look away.
You take my picture
(not asking even)
for your literary magazine
or rock video
or newspaper.
I hope you remember
my face
because you don't
remember me.

You say "Get help!"
But where?
I've been in six states
only seen ten shelters
but hundreds of homeless.
You say I dirty your streets.
You always cross them
to avoid me.

You say I drink too much,
talk to the air.
I don't!
I don't drink
I don't do drugs
and I don't sleep.
Could you out here?

It may be cold in
the winter
but I think
it's colder
in people's hearts.
If you see
someone
talk to the air
maybe
they talk to God.
It sounds crazy to you
because you don't really listen
or see.
You have never lived
on the streets.
I've been homeless
six months this year,
it isn't the first time.
My voice started out quiet
became weak
became congested.
I listen to the sky
(sometimes I reach out
to hug it).
I understand the air
the seduction of the wind
the fear of a lightning storm
the evening hour
and midnight.
I don't talk to it (yet);
I listen to it.
I talk to you
I write to you
of homelessness

in the American Dream
(Ha! Illusions!)
turned nightmare.
I'll keep writing, talking, screaming;
you can't silence me.
I refuse to be
a refugee in my own country.

And you
call me mentally ill.
Why?
Because I'm homeless?
I'm no more
"mentally ill"
than my country is.
So take my picture;
forget my face.
I am a part of
society's disgrace.
Remember my words
my voice
our voices
individuals
in an international
illusion/crisis.
We talk to the air
because we can't
find you anywhere.

WHY *SHOULD* THE POOR ALWAYS BE WITH US?[*]

Angela Browne

Nobody asks the *right* questions. Like thousands of other "survivors" before him, Gary died by his own hand—miserable, frightened, and poor. It was only last summer that I helped facilitate an attempt on his part to sue the company that manufactured Prozac.[**] Gary was certain the drug caused him to experience a severe form of mania, to spend all of his money and allow his credit bills to pile up to an unmanageable portion of his meager income. Following this "manic phase," which appeared to be the first episode he ever experienced, he descended into a deep depression. He approached his fourth floor balcony after a slight altercation with his girlfriend and he jumped. He was later pronounced dead at the hospital, as a result of severe blood loss and brain damage resultant from broken bones and a crushed skull. The news registered in my

---

[*] The author notes that the opinions expressed in this article are her own and do not necessarily reflect the activities of her business, the membership of any organizations, government departments, or other people directly implicated or named. The facts presented here are derived from her experiences on the boards of several psychiatric survivor and mental-health-related organizations in Ontario.

[**] Prozac is a relatively new antidepressant with a controversial history with respect to its relationship to exacerbating suicidal impulses and other forms of psychological distress in some people. There have been a few lawsuits in the United States that have blamed the drug for numerous acts of sudden, unexplained violence, and psychotic behavior.

brain on a cold, sour note, as I cynically remembered the days of yesterday when I still had some fight left in me.

This time, when I heard the news, I picked up my pillow, turned over in bed, and did not go to work that day. I had nothing left to share. The words to an old Bob Dylan song came to mind after so many years: "How many deaths will it take 'til he knows that too many people have died?" Gary's girlfriend Melinda, who was subsequently hospitalized for her own grief reaction to his death, confided that Gary had frequently been depressed as a result of being poor, labeled "unemployable," and kept out of the workforce.

I, for one, can only relate *too* well. Before I managed to secure some ongoing financial support through my own business, I lived through twelve years of intermittent welfare dependency and low-paid employment. As a psychiatric survivor, I struggled through the expected prejudices of a middle-class, mentalist society that expected me to find satisfaction through unpaid, volunteer work or dull, minimum-wage labor. Although I discontinued any direct treatment in the mental health system approximately six years ago, I became "processed" in a seemingly brand new way. As the psychiatric survivor movement, we were *almost* fooled—even though *some* of us still are, by some of the imposed solutions by government and service providers once again.

As recently as five years ago, the province of Ontario was going through what was referred to as "mental health reform," where the latest political buzzwords were *empowerment* and *consumer participation*. The academic press was showered with references to a "new" way of doing things in the mental health system, which included actually *listening* to "consumers"* of the mental health system, putting them into decision-making roles on the boards and staff of mental health agencies, and funding

---

* The term *consumer* is not preferred by the author. To be a consumer of any service, one must be in a position to seek and receive these services voluntarily, as well as be able to choose from a number of competing options. Furthermore, "consumers" have the absolute right to refuse to use certain products and services if they find them to be unacceptable. This is not true with mental health services, where there are few choices and such services are often imposed involuntarily.

a few "consumer" groups.* This was a trend that symbolized for many the latest attempt to coopt what was fast becoming a strong, cohesive psychiatric survivor *movement.*

While the provincial movement was striving to gain for survivors more control over their own lives, access to employment and income, access to meaningful relationships, as well as dignity and self-respect, these goals were being slowly undermined by a mountain of bureaucracy and powerful economic interests. However, as people in the movement are quickly learning, theories do not feed empty stomachs, release people who are now being abused, or bring about the kind of changes we need to make this world a better place to live. Vast differences exist between perspectives in the ivory tower of mental health reform and the actual realities faced every day by psychiatric survivors.

For most Canadian mental health workers of the middle class, *life goes on* under "mental health reform." They drive to work, pretend they care about the homeless, the pro-choice movement, animal liberation, or whatever cause is *in* this month. (Is it *not* the social charter for economic reform *this* month, or was that *last* month?) Catching up on politically correct (PC) talk, the middle-class flock to conferences that are often held far from public transit, pay their $50 registration fees, and pretend to be *pro*-empowerment. Some of the more alert providers have noted the lack of "consumers" at these conferences, while others assume "consumers" are simply not interested. While many of these people *do* care, most cannot fight the latest trend in bureaucratization and continued interests of the status quo. As they continue to replicate PC motivations and behaviors, the duplicity of enforcing the "medical model" under the guise of the "empowerment" model becomes less clear to the most

---

* Examples of documents referring to this new order include *From Consumer to Citizen* (Church, 1986), *Listening to People who Have Directly Experienced the Mental Health System* (Hutchison, Lord, Savage, & Schnarr, 1985), *Consumer Participation: From Concept to Reality* (Pape, 1985), *Participating with People who Have Directly Experienced the Mental Health System* (Hutchison, Lord, & Osborne-Way, 1986), *A Framework for Support for People with Severe Mental Disabilities* (Trainor & Church, 1984). All of the above are published through the Canadian Mental Health Association in Toronto, Ontario.

vulnerable among us. This results in apparently "liberal"
motivations on the part of service providers, while reasons for
the tragedies of the inner city are quietly explained away. As
interest grows for getting more "consumers" on so-called
volunteer boards and committees of mental health bodies to tell
providers what "consumers" want, their prerequisite
pipedreams about a bigger, more expensive mental health system
are sadly becoming more and more of a reality.

▲ ▲ ▲

As middle-class service providers continue to solidify their
ongoing debates about how to liberalize their agency boards to
make them more consumer-friendly, the Ozanam Centre and
City Mission are packed at mealtimes with lonely, shattered
minds.

Paul sits quietly in the corner closing his eyes and dozing off.
While seemingly at peace on this day, he had gone through a
long night. It is hard to find a safe place in a mass of pavement,
cement, and steel. The cold, crisp February air forced him to
remain on his feet, wandering from doughnut shop to doughnut
shop, hoping the managers do not enforce what appears to be
a thirty-minute limit to "customer" patronage. As he left his last
doughnut shop, the doors of the soup kitchen opened. In here,
Paul could catch some shut-eye before he is once again forced
out to find another spot to rest his weary, tired body.

Jennifer pulled on her sweater, complaining of the cold.
Community Care, a local charity that provides food and
clothing to the city's destitute, did not have a coat her size this
month. Jennifer was forced to make do with a heavy sweater
that appears to be a size or two too small for her. As Paul opened
his eyes, Jennifer casually mentioned the name of a man who
had supposedly died the night before. Like Paul, he was forced
to remain out in the cold when the frost bit the region. As the
cold snow overtook the outside world, he went to sleep in a bus
shelter and did not wake up. Nobody was sure if this man had
a family in the area. This man, like many others, will probably
be buried in an unmarked grave paid for by the municipal
welfare department.

Rolande quietly counted his change in his wallet, as he
explained the difficulties he had in cashing his welfare cheque
at a local Money Mart. As usual, the preceding week before
check day seemed to be too difficult for Rolande to wait

through, so he opted for the decreased allotment he received by cashing his cheque early at the local Money Mart.

In the meantime, the conference folks were busy listening to a seminar on mental health planning and model development. Because Virginia is employed as a program director at a local mental health agency, her attendance at this conference was paid for by her employer. As she consumes another complementary cup of coffee, she carefully notes the progress of the meeting. The facilitator, who stood beside the ubiquitous overhead projector, explains to the audience how decreased funding to institutions (or what is euphemistically referred to as "deinstitutionalization") somehow caused homelessness and increased criminal activity among psychiatric patients. The speaker, who was employed as a department head at a nearby psychiatric facility and claimed to have no conflicts of interest in his approach to model development, advocated a more gradual approach to community mental health planning and a strong role for institutional sector involvement. As he stated, trade unions were displeased as governments cut hospital budgets by untold millions, while community mental health agencies visibly competed for what few dollars remained after scarce public funds were squeezed through a fiscal belt-tightening exercise. In a last ditch effort, academics and department heads of major psychiatric facilities argue that an association exists between the horrors of the inner city and deinstitutionalization. However, it does not matter that such theories seem to be more popular as hospitals are forced to close more beds and cut staff.

Arguments for and against deinstitutionalization are merely academic exercises, while the people who are directly affected continue to be transformed into statistics and bureaucratization heads up the battle for political correctness and agency empire-building. As the conference drew to a close, a second part to the series was planned for the following week in a nearby city. At this point, nobody realized the city in which the second part of the conference was planned was without public transportation or that it was to take place in an inaccessible building. Among those present, nobody complained about the time or place. All of those present were able to attend. Ironically, the topic of the next workshop was the role of the "consumer" in mental health planning. In spite of what resulted in copious discussion with respect to how to involve "consumers" in this workshop, it was obvious that most (if not all) "consumers" would not be there on that day either.

In the local mental health drop-in centre, Mary put out her smoking cigarette butt and opened a two-day-old newspaper to the classified ads. In the background, the usual rumble of euchre and television competed for an audience against the rough and tumble of two fellows arguing over who owed whom a package of cigarettes. With at least another fortnight to go until their disability checks arrived, the addicted become desperate. The night before, there had been a burglary at the drop-in center. Robert, the person responsible for this burglary, broke into staff filing cabinets where cigarettes and petty cash were kept. The police arrived at the drop-in centre early in the morning and took Robert into custody. As usual, the minds of other members who were present and heard the news about Robert quickly returned to their comfortable routines of euchre and television soap operas. Powerlessness overcomes the will to question what has now become a routine matter in the lives of many.

In the minds of the middle-class, local churches and charities do their bit. Many denominations give people a place to stay for a few nights, something to eat, a place to play cards, and to wander around. In the minds of those numbed by this desperate existence, churches provide *necessities* for them in return for a bit of prayer, as well as personal pride. Many will keep on praying in hopes their circumstances will improve or return to their former level of prosperity. In return, the members of the community feel they have done their share, even though the actual number of people living in poverty seems to be increasing with the passage of time. In the minds of true believers, Jesus will return some day to restore prosperity and hope in the lives of the desperate, but nobody ever offers solutions in the meantime. In the meantime, Mary falls asleep on the couch with the newspaper folded out on her lap.

In the city of Fort Erie, where the second part of the mental health conference was held, the guest speaker pointed to a screen full of numbers and in bureaucratese tried to explain why the money failed to follow patients into the community. It seemed that while more and more people were moving out of the institutions, more *money* was getting poured into them. This speaker, who was considerably more progressive than the previous week's speaker, proposed a model where resources could be more evenly distributed and more people referred to as major stakeholders could have more say in how the pie is cut. It is no longer PC to exclude "consumers"—in principle anyway.

During a scheduled break period, Virginia glanced at a newspaper and noticed an ad for the position of a *half-time* Social Worker at a nearby hospital for $37,500 a year.[*] As with most institutionally-based positions, this job paid just a little more than her current full-time position as a community-based mental health worker. So much for deinstitutionalization. While life goes on for the middle-class conference participants, a few people continued to cry alone.

Melinda, the girlfriend Gary left behind in his successful suicide bid, noticed there was no food in her cupboard. Desperate for something else to fill her void, she went crazy. She wanted her friend back, the one who passed away. Melinda knew that, at least in part, his death was precipitated by the dreadful poverty, the painful drudgery of emptiness, having nowhere to go, nothing to do, and nothing to live for except the day of his next disability check. The magnitude of personal suffering is big when somebody close to you dies. Nothing could replace the shadow that stood in her doorway when she needed his comforting, his personal warmth and tenderness that helped her return to reality when she had flashbacks about her own personal experiences of sexual abuse as a young child, a shoulder to cry on when nobody else in the world appeared to care about her pain and her existence. Her only sense of comfort was gone. Melinda's sense of happiness followed her friend to his grave.

As the conference wrapped up, this "ivory tower" version of reality continued to ignore basic facts that were only too clear to the experiences of Paul, Jennifer, Rolande, Gary, Mary, Melinda, and the majority of psychiatric survivors attempting to make their way in the so-called community these days. First, virtually everybody knows that mental disorder is tied to poverty. Moreover, significant numbers of "survivors" are unemployed, living on less than $10,000 a year, and often have to resort to food banks and soup kitchens for bare essentials.[**] Furthermore, the association between poverty, unemployment,

---

[*] This was actually an advertised position brought to my attention by a psychiatric survivor living in the Niagara region.

[**] D. Ross & R. Shillington, *An Economic Profile of Persons with Disabilities in Canada* (Ottawa: Secretary of State, 1990).

and even poorer mental health is clear.[*] As people descend into resultant psychiatric crisis, the increased use of expensive hospital services is obvious. Therefore, everybody knows that deinstitutionalization does not save the government a dime. It simply moved the attitudes that were inherent in the institution back into the community, where personal suffering and tragedy are allowed to continue.

▲ ▲ ▲

In 1991, provincial bureaucrats and mental health workers began to redesign psychiatric institutions and traditional services to look like our "community" will be getting a break at last. They allocated $3.7 million from the Ministry of Health specifically for the funding of several local, regional, and provincial organizations of psychiatric survivors. In response, groups of psychiatric survivors were granted funding under this program and began organizing in their respective communities to make changes. The steering committee of the provincial Ontario Psychiatric Survivors Alliance (OPSA) was enthusiastic, perhaps mistakenly, about these new initiatives. When the psychiatric survivor movement gained strength in Ontario, funding decisions were ultimately used in an attempt to stagnate our growth and development.

In its own unusual way, this provincial initiative served as an impetus to further expose the thinly disguised agenda of institutional psychiatry and the mental health system. This cleverly designed scheme, while appearing to be progressive, reinforced the status quo of institutional power and control.

First, the attitude that psychiatric survivors *could not* or *should not* be in the paid labor force was prevalent, even though superficially these projects supported the opposite. Among thousands of psychiatric survivors who were out of work and in need of paid employment, only a small handful were hired by the projects. Initially, movement activists believed they would be getting most of the paid work, but this dream soon diminished. Among those who did find and maintain this employment over time, only a few had significant organizational development

---

[*] R. Warner, *Recovery from Schizophrenia: Psychiatry and Political Economy* (New York: Routledge & Kegan Paul, 1985).

experience. Though some of the projects focused on economic development and providing paid work to additional psychiatric survivors through the creation of small businesses, most of these jobs were low paying, low skilled and, often, only used to supplement monthly disability benefits rather than replace them. With an economy as poor as it is in Ontario, the excuse of having only so much money to go around is believable. When assessing the impact of this new funding, it is more vital to examine what happened to people who were not paid but who were in fact marginalized through its development and how the potentially vulnerable survivors were successfully used to continue this process by shutting out their own predecessors.

Second, the attitude that psychiatric survivors were incapable of helping themselves and managing their own organizations was prevalent. Once again, the superficial message was that this initiative was "empowering" to people and that for the first time disempowered people were taking back their power and managing their own lives and organizations. However, under the guise of appearing liberal and flexible to funded groups, the Ministry developed few policies to govern how this funding was to be used. While having few policies *can* open the doors to funded groups having the freedom to develop their programs and policies in the way they felt most comfortable, this "liberalism" can be horrific. This so-called "flexibility" worked both ways. While some groups were able to take advantage of this flexibility, others became subject to unchecked power and control over their agenda by the funder. Where there were no policies dictating what each funded organization can do with its funding, there were no policies protecting organizations from abuse by their funders either.

Third, the attitude that psychiatric survivors have no right to become political is prevalent. On paper it appears the funders do not wish to control an organization's political agenda. However, as the founders of the Ontario Psychiatric Survivors Alliance were gradually isolated by newly active survivors in their own regions, it became only too clear our own political agenda was not acceptable to the Ministry either. The attitude that we *cannot* or *should not* get political is painfully relevant. We were not to question the use of medication, the "medical model," the function of ordinarily well paid service providers, or, least of all, the motivations of the funder. We are further expected to accept implausible explanations as to why our people continue to be so miserable. Under the guise of promoting "open democracy" among survivor members of the Ontario Psychiatric Survivors Alliance, we were discouraged from taking strong stands against the system. In October 1992, we were advised by Ministry officials that OPSA would be receiving $300,000 per year, down from our previous allotment of $450,000 per year. Prior to or simultaneous to the meeting in which we were advised of this decision, several local funded groups were offered extra money to do regional development. This appeared to be a thinly veiled attempt to trap OPSA to compete against local groups so that its credibility would quickly decline, thereby providing an excuse for the Ministry to completely cut the remaining funds allocated to OPSA.

This method of "divide and conquer" could easily be achieved, given the nearly universal situation of poverty among psychiatric survivors. We have found that those with jobs under the projects were less accepting of OPSA and were easily manipulated into acting to overthrow their own local boards. There have been reported cases of project staff receiving instruction from representatives of the Ministry of Health to breach their board's confidentiality provisions as well as directives to set up unethical membership recruitment processes and to even close up shop in one case! Because many of these paid employees lack the self-confidence or educational qualifications necessary to seek work elsewhere, they may have been reluctant to challenge such directives. Little has been publicly stated about these abuses, but they have been well documented by activists in the survivor movement.

Instead of directly alleviating the universal state of poverty among psychiatric survivors, this process perpetuated it. The public seems convinced that poverty among psychiatric survivors has been alleviated, yet poverty, dependency on social assistance, and personal trauma continue for the majority of psychiatric survivors. But this time our suffering has been made invisible.

We know of several cases of psychiatric survivors becoming isolated from their local groups, psychiatric survivors becoming hospitalized, and even a few suicides. One suicide occurred in a psychiatric survivor who started off devoted to the original dream of the movement in his region. When these dreams failed to turn into reality, he was used in a successful "board takeover" and was later reported dead, with the cause of death listed as suicide. Our apparent failure to conform to other people's agendas will only be used to demonstrate that psychiatric survivors *cannot* work, *cannot* run their own organizations, *cannot* make appropriate decisions about their lives, and *cannot* articulate their own needs. This will ultimately provide an opening for service providers and institutions to move in and take over where our movement left off.

The results of this funding initiative certainly differ from its originally stated intent. Though I cannot comment on real or hidden intents of those persons responsible for administering the Ministry of Health funding, these problems appear to be continuing as though these results were acceptable. Once again, we risk accusations that we have merely imagined our abuse, our suffering, and resultant cooptation. These accusations are only too familiar for those among us who experienced sexual and other forms of abuse but were not listened to by those who should have listened.

Abuse continues to occur in all psychiatric institutions as well as in the community. The fact that a large percentage of psychiatric survivors is out of work (and most of them live on incomes below $10,000) shows that this kind of lifestyle continues to be some kind of acceptable standard. The continued ignorance and lack of effort toward resolving these issues continues to condemn a very large number of psychiatric survivors to living on permanent disability pensions. Most of them are told, in spite of their skills and educational attainment, they can never become productive citizens again.

Long-term dependence on disability benefits destroys one's ability to maintain structure to one's day, make meaningful social contacts and become involved in long-term relationships. Furthermore, administration of social benefits in itself discourages employment or even receipt of other forms of independent income. However, despite all of this, many psychiatric survivors wish to become employed and leave the social assistance system. When this funding started, many of us were hopeful because these jobs paid as much as or even more than the average salary of mental health workers. In the competition for these jobs, many survivors were ambivalent about applying because they were concerned that after these jobs ended they would have no income from employment, disability benefits, or otherwise. As a result, most of the survivors receiving social assistance at all, who eventually became employed by these jobs, were *not* originally on disability benefits. They tended to be on unemployment insurance, general welfare assistance, or "mothers allowance" (Canadian social benefits used to assist single parents). This attitude simply reinforced the myth that people on disability benefits cannot work, and therefore should not be entitled to work. While this initiative continued to pit survivors against survivors, proponents of this Ministry of Health program continued to use creative marketing of assembled statistics to "prove" their funding was working, as people were supposedly using expensive hospital services less, and leaving the rolls of social assistance. The problems inherent in research design and the statistical methods used to generate these figures are too complex to explain here, but if proper controls were put into place when these surveys were first carried out the program would be unlikely to demonstrate the positive results that were touted across the province.

Finally, the invisibility of the real problems faced on a day-to-day basis by psychiatric survivors has further trivialized the deaths of our brothers and sisters. While the powers that be continue to blame these deaths on the purported pathology in these individuals and not the community that has incarcerated them into a cruel lifestyle, these concerns will continue. Popular misconceptions continue to include the supposed "fact" that the psychiatric "survivors" in question "went off" their medication or did not bother to seek "appropriate" help. It continues to be the victim's fault, no matter how obviously outside circumstances appeared to contribute to a person's demise.

Robert, one of the persons described above, recently died of a heart attack. He was no more than 40 years of age. Mary, also described above, recently had a liaison with another person in the drop-in center mentioned earlier. A few months ago, Mary was found dead in her apartment. The cause of her death was murder. Paul has disappeared and no one has been able to locate him for more than two months. The "rumor mill" depicts Paul as having left to look for work in Milton. When someone tried to reach Paul, there was no listing for him in Milton, nor does anybody we spoke to in Milton know of Paul's whereabouts. I saw Jennifer two weeks ago at the soup kitchen. She told me she had been raped by her landlord. Of course, Jennifer did not pursue any charges against him, as she is unable to find another place to live so cheaply in the region. Besides that, who would believe her, anyway? Rolande, the fellow depicted above as having used Money Mart to cash his welfare checks, was sentenced to a jail term for breaking and entering into a church when he was unable to find a place to sleep one recent cold February night.

While I can only speak for people in the Niagara region, my contacts in the survivor movement are telling similar stories across Ontario. While Rolande can be assured of having enough to eat and a bed to sleep in for a short period of time, he cannot be assured he will ever become "empowered" under the new mental health reform project, as defined by service providers and bureaucrats who continue to be so out of touch with our real needs.

In the meantime—in middle-class suburbia, Virginia has applied for the $37,500 per year social work position at the nearby psychiatric facility. After all, Virginia knows all the hype around "deinstitutionalization" is particularly cosmetic. Virginia knows that in the mental health world, the higher the position in which one is employed and the more money they make, the less they need to see of real psychiatric survivors. Therefore, under the new rules set by what appears to be the latest code for political correctness, the ladder of achievement and success is measured by the degree to which one can remain out of touch with the real needs of psychiatric survivors yet remain so damned sympathetic. So much for illusions about changing the system. A few years from now, Virginia will attend another one of those conferences, except it will be her this time—the facilitator standing beside the ubiquitous overhead projector, outlining ways in which "consumers" of the mental health system can become meaningfully involved in designing the mental health system of the future. As long as we allow this to continue, the new model for mental health planning will always be comparable to simply rearranging the chairs on the deck of the Titanic, while only providing a better view for all the supposed stakeholders while going down!

▲ ▲ ▲

While I do not disapprove of the government funding psychiatric survivor groups in themselves, as these resources can and have gone a long way toward development of the survivor movement and have potential for reaching a very large segment of our population, such funding should not be tied at all to the political motivation of service providers, institutional interests, or government bureaucrats. Furthermore, funding set out with a primary purpose of employing psychiatric survivors should only be tied to large-scale economic development and full utilization of talents, skills, and experience of psychiatric survivors, both as the psychiatric survivors themselves see fit and as the private market will dictate. Long-term employment and reduction in the use of social benefits will not come about as a result of publicly funded positions alone, nor will it come about through the use of funded psychiatric survivor groups alone—although both methods will yield a few good jobs for survivors who might not ordinarily have them.

Continued marginalization and isolation of psychiatric survivors by funders, service providers, and the survivor community is a poor way to use potential talent that rests in these people. Opportunities should be made available for removing as many psychiatric survivors as possible from the rolls of disability benefits, as well as other forms of social assistance. This should be a priority, particularly with those psychiatric survivors who wish to become meaningfully employed. This cannot be done by providing high-paying jobs for only a handful of psychiatric survivors; it requires the use of community economic development techniques that will make it not only possible but profitable for psychiatric survivors—alone or in groups—to start their own businesses, work for private sector employers, and help other psychiatric survivors in obtaining long-term, full-time employment. The positive impact of employment on the lives of psychiatric survivors is clear.

One critique of affirmative action is that many of its beneficiaries lack the necessary qualifications to do the job and appear to be hired solely on the basis of their membership in a minority group. I do not support this approach to affirmative action, because it can lead to reverse discrimination. Psychiatric survivors, like anybody else, should be employed in fields in which they have both educational and experiential qualifications. A more positive approach to affirmative action is first to assist psychiatric survivors in obtaining these necessary qualifications and then to assist them in finding employment. Any affirmative action program should include entrepreneurship, self-employment, and professional work opportunities as options, in addition to placements with existing employers.

Programs that assist psychiatric survivors in starting their own businesses or provide them with necessary funds under special loan programs will go a long way toward getting many psychiatric survivors employed without spending massive amounts of public money. Assistance in obtaining and maintaining a good credit rating is essential to continuing and expanding a business, so government might provide some regulatory and program assistance in these areas to psychiatric survivors who demonstrate positive potential. Furthermore, governments should also encourage the development and growth of such businesses. Finally, access to postsecondary education and training should be made readily available to psychiatric survivors who wish to be employed in fields that normally require these qualifications in nonsurvivors.

How can government policymakers encourage this to happen? First, government departments sometimes contract work to the private sector. These tasks vary in the degree of skill and training required as much as they do in the private sector. These tasks include construction and contracting, application of skilled trades, secretarial and clerical services, technical research services, consulting services, management services, community development services, catering services, and many other kinds of services. Nonprofit organizations funded by government sources often ask their funders to suggest a list of providers in their area that could carry out these kinds of specialized tasks for their organizations. Among the psychiatric survivor community, there are many people with the necessary skills and training to carry out these tasks as well as, or perhaps even better than, their non-psychiatric-survivor competitors. Along with the development of psychiatric survivor-run businesses and appropriate affirmative action guidelines for other private sector suppliers, businesses that are run by and/or employ psychiatric survivors with appropriate qualifications should be given priority when contracts are being handed out or referrals are made. Ongoing support and consultation should be made available to such businesses through economic development councils set up for each region. Assistance with accommodation issues can be done both on a private consultation basis and through public education efforts of psychiatric survivor organizations that have a successful track record in dealing with employment accommodation.

Social benefits legislation must be changed to encourage its beneficiaries to find employment. When a person works, her or his social benefits are often taxed back as much as 100 percent of the amount of monies earned through paid employment. This policy must end immediately, as this provides no financial incentive for recipients of social benefits to find paid work. While taking the costs associated with working, social benefits legislation should tax benefits only to the extent that a person's total net monthly income exceeds the amount they would otherwise have received from social benefits alone. The amount by which the person's total monthly income exceeds social benefit levels when working must increase as more money is earned by paid employment. This will provide a financial incentive to those who would otherwise be "trapped" on social benefits.

Differential treatment for "employable" and "unemployable" persons on social assistance must end, in favor of social benefits that deliver income maintenance on the basis of need and cost of living alone, with additional support to those persons whose needs are greater. When I conducted interviews for my study on disability benefits, many people stated their doctors or social workers told them they were unable to work, and therefore they qualified for the higher level of benefits. Psychiatric survivors as a group tend to lack self-confidence as it is, without being told by people in authority they cannot work again (for which proof of "unemployability" is once again subject to interpretation).

Finally, mental health services delivered to psychiatric survivors must be sensitive to the necessity of normalization in their lives. Most psychiatric rehabilitation models encourage survivors to become full time patients or clients to such an extent that they cannot fit paid employment into their rehabilitation schedules. Such rehabilitation and mental health services should only be delivered voluntarily to people who wish to use them, and such programs should have built-in financial incentives to produce positive changes in the lives of people they serve. Having psychiatric survivors on their boards as a mandatory component of their funding is just part of the solution. Such services should only be funded in accordance with the number of people who voluntarily use them as well as benefit from them. For example, if such a program promises its users they will find employment at the end of it, the program will be funded in accordance with the number of people voluntarily using it and actually finding work after they finish. If such a program proves useless in helping people achieve employment goals, and people do not wish to use it, the agency responsible for administering such a program should have its financial security put into jeopardy—unless it meets guidelines for correction within a prescribed period of time. Naturally, it is not possible for any program to find employment for all of its users, but particular standards must continue to be met. If these solutions and recommendations were put into place by any government in the Western world, the amount of unemployment among psychiatric survivors would certainly decrease significantly. Increased welfare rates will not necessarily or even probably end poverty; the solution for eliminating poverty rests with full employment. With an increase in the number of psychiatric survivors employed, a subsequent drop in their poverty rates will follow.

Appendix A

Organizations and Publications for Psychiatric Survivors

Altered States of the Arts

c/o Gayle Bluebird, 110 SW 8th Ave., Ft. Lauderdale, FL 33312

Altered States of the Arts is an organization of psychiatric survivor artists, writers and performers who promote political awareness and change through the arts. They put out *The Altered State*, a quarterly publication of survivors' works. They also organize displays and performances at conferences and events.

The Committee For Truth In Psychiatry

P.O. Box 1214, New York, NY 10003

Founded by the late Marilyn Rice, CTIP is an organization of former shock patients who advocate for the adoption of laws and regulations that would require psychiatrists to give prospective shock patients truthful information about the procedure and its effects.

Dendron

P.O. Box 11284, Eugene, OR 97440

Dendron is an outstanding newspaper that reaches thousands of psychiatric survivors internationally. Founded and edited by David Oakes, it is packed with information: news on resources and survivor/consumer groups; articles about psychiatric oppression, the survivor movement, alternatives to psychiatric treatment;

announcements of upcoming events; humor; news items nationwide and abroad. Very highly recommended. Annual subscription rates: $10.00 for individuals; $20.00 for institutions.

National Association of Protection and Advocacy Systems
220 Eye Street N.E., Suite 150, Washington D.C., 20001
Phone 202-546-8202

If you have been or are being abused by psychiatric treatment and wish to obtain legal aid, NAPAS will put you in contact with advocacy agencies in your area.

National Association For Rights Protection and Advocacy
587 Marshall Ave., St. Paul, MN 55102

NARPA is made up of survivors, lawyers, mental health professionals and other individuals who advocate for patients' rights. They publish a newsletter, *The Rights Tenet*, which includes reports from The Center For the Study of Psychiatry. Founded by Peter Breggin, CSP is a research/educational group which studies current psychiatric trends and works for psychiatric reform. NARPA also holds an annual convention on patients' rights and psychiatric reform.

National Directory of Mental Health Consumers, Expatients, Organizations, & Resources
SC SHARE, 722 Blanding St., Columbia, SC 29201;
1-800-832-8032

This directory, published by the South Carolina Self-Help Association, consists of 100 pages of consumer run/self-help groups.

National Empowerment Center
130 Parker St., Suite 20, Lawrence, MA 01843

NEC is a federally-funded project with centers in Massachusetts and Pennsylvania. They hold monthly teleconferences where psychiatric survivor leaders discuss preannounced topics. Tapes of these conferences can be obtained from NEC. NEC also runs the annual Alternatives conference and tapes of conference

workshops are also available. NEC has put together a list
of consumer/expatient survivor-run groups throughout
the U.S. for networking and referrals. To get on their
mailing list and receive their newsletter, call them
toll-free at 1-800-POWER-2-U.

International Resources

Disabled Persons International
101-7 Evergreen Place, Winnipeg, Manitoba,
Canada R3L 2Y3

A cross-disability coalition of self-help organizations of
people in 90 countries.

Psychiatric Survivor Network in Canada
Ontario Psychiatric Survivors Alliance, 3107 Bloor Street
West, Suite 207, Etobicoke, Ontario M8X 1E3 Canada.

Psychiatric Survivor Network in New Zealand
Aotearoa Network of Psychiatric Survivors, P.O. Box
46-018 Herne Bay, Auckland, New Zealand.

Psychiatric Survivor Network in England
MIND, 22 Harley Street, London W1N 2ED England.

Support Coalition International
S.C.I. co-coordinator Janet Foner, 920 Brandt Ave., New
Cumberland, PA 17070; 717-774-6465; Email:
janetfon@aol.com

Support Coalition International main office, David Oakes,
P.O. Box 11284, Eugene, OR 97440; 503-341-0100; Email:
chrp@enf.org

An alliance of sponsoring groups concerned about
human rights in and alternatives to psychiatry.

World Federation of Psychiatric Users

Mary O'Hagan—Chairperson WFPU, c/o Center For
Mental Health Services Development, King's College,
Campden Hill Rd., London W8 7AH England

The World Federation of Psychiatric Users is an
international networking group which has recently
formed with centers in Japan, England, Wales, Mexico,
the Netherlands, U.S.A. and New Zealand. It connects
ex-patients, consumers, survivors, users and clients
throughout the world in their common goals.

Appendix B

Suggested Reading

This book list was compiled, in part, through a questionnaire sent to the contributors asking what books they would recommend to other women survivors to aid in their empowerment.

Anthologies and Collections by Survivors and Consumers

Browne, Susan E., Debra Connors and Nanci Stern, eds. *With the Power of Each Breath: A Disabled Women's Anthology.* San Francisco: Cleis Press, 1985.

Burstow, Bonnie, and Don Weitz, eds. *Shrink Resistant: The Struggle Against Psychiatry in Canada.* Vancouver: New Star Publications, 1988.

Geller, Jeffrey L. and Maxine Harris. *Women of the Asylum: Voices from Behinds the Walls, 1840-1945.* New York: Anchor Books, 1994.

Hirsch, Sherry, et al, eds. *Madness Network News Reader.* San Francisco: Glide Publications, 1974.

Howe, Florence, and Marsha Saxton, eds. *With Wings: An Anthology of Literature By and About Women With Disabilities.* New York: The Feminist Press, 1987.

Oakes, John G. H., ed. *In the Realms of the Unreal: "Insane" Writings.* New York: Four Walls Eight Windows, 1991.

Sinister Wisdom 36: Surviving Psychiatric Assault & Creating Emotional Well-Being in Our Communities. Winter 1988/89 Issue. Sinister Wisdom, P.O. Box 3252, Berkeley, CA 94703.

Susko, Michael A., ed. *Cry of the Invisible: Writings From the Homeless and Survivors of Psychiatric Hospitals.* Baltimore: The Conservatory Press, 1991.

Books by Survivors and Consumers

Blackbridge, Persimmon and Sheila Gilhooly. *Still Sane.* Vancouver, Canada: Press Gang Publishers, 1989.

Erickson, Elaine. *Solo Drive.* Baltimore: Chestnut Hills Press, 1992.

Farmer, Frances. *Will There Really Be a Morning?* New York: Dell, 1972.

Frame, Janet. *Faces in the Water.* 1961; reprint. New York: George Braziller, Inc., 1982.

Freeman, Huey. *Judge, Jury and Executioner.* Urbana, IL: Talking Leaves Press, 1986.

Greally, Hanna. *Bird's Nest Soup.* Dublin, Ireland: Attic Press, 1971.

Gotkin, Janet, and Paul Gotkin. *Too Much Anger, Too Many Tears: A Personal Triumph Over Psychiatry.* 1975; reprint. New York: Harper Perennial, 1992.

Kaysen, Susanna. *Girl, Interrupted.* New York: Turtle Bay Books, 1993.

Millett, Kate. *The Loony Bin Trip.* New York: Simon & Schuster, 1990.

Plath, Sylvia. *The Bell Jar.* New York: Harper and Row, 1971.

Supeene, Shelagh Lynne. *As For the Sky Falling: A Critical Look at Psychiatry and Suffering.* Toronto, Canada: Second Story Press, 1990.

Weinbaum, Batya. *The Island of Floating Women.* San Diego: Clothespin Fever Press, 1993.

Critical Works Challenging Psychiatry and the Mental Health System

Armstrong, Louise. *And They Call It Help: The Psychiatric Policing of America's Children.* Reading, MA: Addison-Wesley, 1993.

Breggin, Peter. *Electroshock: Its Brain-Disabling Effects.* New York: Springer, 1979.

Breggin, Peter, M.D., and Ginger Ross Breggin. *Talking Back to Prozac: What Doctors Aren't Telling You About Today's Most Controversial Drug.* NewYork: St. Martin's Press, 1994.

Breggin, Peter. *Toxic Psychiatry.* New York: St. Martin's Press, 1991.

Breggin, Peter, M.D., and Ginger Ross Breggin. *The War Against Children: How the Drugs, Programs and Theories of the Psychiatric Establishment Are Threatening America's Children With a Medical "Cure" for Violence.* New York: St. Martin's Press, 1994.

Caplan, Paula J. *They Say You're Crazy.* Reading, MA: Addison-Wesley, 1995.

Chamberlin, Judi. *On Our Own: Patient-Controlled Alternatives to the Mental Health System.* New York, 1978; reprint. London: MIND, 1993. For Ordering information, write to MIND Consumer Network, 22 Harley St., London W1N 2ED England.

Chesler, Phyllis. *Women and Madness.* New York: Harcourt Brace Jovanovich, 1989.

Cohen, David, ed. *Challenging the Therapeutic State: Critical Perspectives on Psychiatry and the Mental Health System.* New York: Institute of Mind and Behavior Press, 1990. For ordering information, write to *Journal,* P.O. Box 522, Village Station, New York, NY 10014.

Cohen, David, ed., *Challenging the Therapeutic State, Part 2: Further Disquisitions on the Mental Health System.* Montreal: University of Montreal: 1994.

Colbert, Ty C., Ph.D. *Depression and Mania: Friends or Foes—A New "Non-Drug" Model of Hope For Depression, Mania and Compulsive Disorders.* Santa Ana, CA: KEVCO Publishers, 1995.

Coleman, Lee. *The Reign of Error: Psychiatry, Authority and Law.* Boston: Beacon Press, 1984.

Ehrenreich, Barbara, and Dierdre English. *Witches, Midwives and Nurses.* New York: Feminist Press, 1963.

Farber, Seth. *Madness, Heresy and the Rumor of Angels: The Revolt Against the Mental Health System.* Peru, Illinois: Open Court, 1993.

Frank, Leonard Roy, ed. *The History of Shock Treatment.* 1978. Available through Leonard Roy Frank, 2300 Webster St., San Francisco, CA 94115.

Heyward, Carter. *When Boundaries Betray Us: Beyond Illusions of What is Ethical in Therapy and Life.* San Francisco: Harper Collins, 1994.

Hillman, James and Michael Ventura. *We've Had a Hundred Years of Psychotherapy (and the World's Only Getting Worse).* New York: Harper San Francisco, 1992.

Kirk, Stuart A. and Herb Kutchins, *The Selling of DSM: The Rhetoric of Science in Psychiatry.* New York: Aldine de Gruyter, 1992.

Laing, R. D. *The Politics of Experience.* New York: Pantheon, 1967.

Lapon, Lenny. *Mass Murderers in White Coats: Psychiatric Genocide in Nazi Germany and the United States.* Springfield, MA: Psychiatric Genocide Research Institute, 1986. Available through The Psychiatric Genocide Research Institute, 55 Bryant St., Springfield, MA 01108.

Lewontin, R. C., Steven Rose and Leon Kamin. *Not In Our Genes.* New York: Pantheon, 1984.

Masson, Jeffrey Moussaieff. *Against Therapy: Emotional Tyranny and the Myth of Psychological Healing.* New York: Atheneum, 1988.

Modrow, John. *How to Become A Schizophrenic: The Case Against Biological Psychiatry.* Apollyon Press, 1992.

Morgan, Robert, ed. *Electroshock: The Case Against.* Toronto: IPI Publishing, 1991.

Mowbray, Carol T., Susan Lanir, and Marilyn Hulce, eds. *Women and Mental Health: New Directions For Change.* Binghamton, NY: Harrington Park Press, 1985.

Smith, Trevor, M.D. *Homeopathic Medicine for Mental Health: A Self-Help Guide to Remedies that Can Restore Calm and Happiness.* Rochester, VT: Healing Arts Press, 1989.

Sharkey, Joe. *Bedlam: Greed, Profiteering, and Fraud in a Mental Health System Gone Crazy.* New York: St. Martin's Press, 1994.

Showalter, Elaine. *The Female Malady: Women, Madness, and English Culture, 1930-1980.* New York: Penguin Books, 1985.

Szasz, Thomas. *Insanity: The Idea and Its Consequences.* New York: John Wiley & Sons, 1987.

Szasz, Thomas. *Law, Liberty and Psychiatry.* New York: Macmillan, 1963.

Szasz, Thomas. *The Manufacture of Madness: A Comparative
   Study of the Inquisition and the Mental Health
   Movement.* 1970; reprint. New York: Harpertorch, 1984.
Szasz, Thomas. *The Myth of Mental Illness: Foundations of a
   Theory of Personal Conduct.* New York: Harper and
   Row, 1974.
Ussher, Jane. *Women's Madness: Misogyny or Mental Illness.*
   Amherst, MA: University of Massachusetts Press, 1992.
Wood, Mary Elene. *The Writing on the Wall: Womens
   Autobiography and the Asylum.* Urbana, IL: University of
   Illinois Press, 1994.

Appendix C

Other Resource Media

Cyberspace

DENDRITE

A one-way human rights message to you from Dendron (see Appendix A for more information about Dendron), about twice a month. To subscribe, send Email to majordomo@enf.org with the sole command: subscribe DENDRITE

MADNESS

A free Internet mailing list for communication with allies, support, and information exchange. Founded by psychiatric survivor Sylvia Caras. To subscribe, send Email to LISTSERV@sjuvm.stjohns.edu with the sole command: subscribe MADNESS yourfirstname yourlastname

HEALNORM

A free Internet mailing list open to anyone who wishes to be part of the Heal Normality Campaign launched by the folks at Support Coalition International. They advertise: "e-mail your creativity to this campaign, such as: warning signs of normality, healing experiences, ideas for normality-transforming pranks & actions." To subscribe, send E-mail to majordomo@enf.org with the sole command: subscribe HEALNORM

Newsletters and Newspapers

Dykes Disability and Stuff
  P.O. Box 8773, Madison, WI 53708-8773

Hikane
  P.O. Box 841, Great Barrington, MA 01230

  Hikane and *Dykes, Disability and Stuff* are both
  excellent newsletters for lesbians with disabilities
  (includes psychiatric disability).

Counterpoint
  RR1, Box 41F, Groton, VT 05046

  Counterpoint is another popular newspaper for
  psychiatric survivors. Highly recommended.

Videotapes

Rainbow Productions. A consumer-run and operated video
  company; reports on consumer affairs; conferences; also,
  interviews, personal stories and educational tapes. For
  complete listing write Rainbow, 24 Farmington St.,
  Chicopee, MA 01020.
Videotape on Feminist Views Against Psychiatry. Write
  Phoenix Rising, 441 Clinton St., Toronto, Ontario, M6G
  2Z1 Canada. (This one is a little expensive—$40.00.)
Videotape on Racist Psychiatry. Available from National
  Public Television. Call 1-800-358-3000. Request
  "Himmler Tape File No. 25."
White Light Communications. Psychiatric Survivor-run video
  company; produces tapes focusing on issues and
  personalities of the Consumer/Survivor Movement. White
  Light Communications, 7 Kilburn St., Burlington, VT
  05401.

About the Contributors

Angela Browne is a university-educated, self-employed psychiatric survivor, community activist, and writer living in St. Catharines, Ontario. Browne has helped found several psychiatric survivor organizations, including the Ontario Psychiatric Survivors Alliance and a local survivor advocacy group. She has a long history of community activism in areas of housing, human rights, anti-poverty issues, economic development, and disability issues. She currently owns and manages Browne Consulting & Research, her own consultation practice, which includes work in organizational development, nonprofit management, and government relations issues.

Angela Hopkins Hart. In the naive early days of jazz criticism, the ultimate accolade was to say that a performer "lived the blues." Angie Hart is like that about surrealism. In her work and in her life, Angie demonstrates the flexibility of apparently rigid structures, the seemingly immutable laws of meaning, and the state apparatus of social control; both assume the malleability of Dali's watches. Stepping through the minefield of proscriptions and prescriptions that make up her own situation tragedy, Angie Hart reveals a viewpoint of authentic difference, instantly familiar and comprehensible to psychic dissidents everywhere.

Anne C. Woodlen describes herself this way: "I am as I appear in the written word. If I sing or weep, roast marshmallows or torture small animals, express great wonder or bore you to tears, I do it all in what I write. The way to know me is to read me: there's the truth of who I am."

Anne Lawton Lunt , poet, painter, percussionist, mother of two members of the Marah Indian Nation, an empowered member of a new human race, is becoming her true self.

Batya Weinbaum still gets depressed but mostly about poverty and bills, and she doubts that's biochemical. Her *Island of*

Floating Women was published by Clothespin Fever Press in 1994 and contains some pretty mystical madness stories.

Beth Greenspan, a 31-year-old poet and observer of life, is dedicated to trying to survive off the beaten path and find peace of mind. Her poetry has been published in journals, newsletters, and anthologies (including *In the Realms of the Unreal: "Insane" Writings*, Four Walls Eight Windows, 1991) across the U.S. Greenspan was employed as an advocate for people in the mental health system for six years and is presently vice president of Pennsylvania Mental Health Consumers' Association. She resides in a supported apartment program with her cat, Kerouac, where together they attempt daily to deal with the overwhelmingness of it all.

Betty Blaska is a psychiatric survivor and an incest survivor. She enjoys activism in the areas of mental health and childhood sexual abuse; cryptograms, anagrams and Scrabble; euchre and table games; and writing. She edits the newsletter *Emerging Force*, the mouthpiece for PREVAIL, Inc. (Psychiatric Reform thru Education, Visionary Action, and Informed Leadership).

Bluebird, 51, is coordinator of Altered States of the Arts, a national organization for artists, writers, and performers who have been through the mental health system. Most recently she was hired by District 10 HRS in Florida to be a Nurse Consultant and Consumer Affairs Coordinator.

Catherine Odette reports "Fifteen years 'inside' almost killed me. Fifteen years after that, I am a survivor. I won, pridefully, a whole slew of labels, which inform my life and politics: I am a disabled, Jewish daughter of Holocaust survivors; a lifelong Lesbian Separatist man-hater; an anti-psychiatry survivor of much of its abuses; a shit-kickin' raised-poor dyke who thinks pain is painful and love is lovely. I have the perfect partner, Sara, and together we work hard to make the world a better place." Publisher-member of a group who put out the only lesbian-only radical disability newsletter *Dykes, Disability & Stuff*, Odette recently completed a collection of works by Jewish lesbian daughters of Holocaust survivors called *The Chosen of The Chosen*, which is still looking for a publisher.

Clover spent thirty-one years being psychiatry's victim, the chronically mentally ill, and accumulated close to fifty psychiatric admissions, always leaving worse off than she entered. (She says the best definition of insanity is said to be the repeating of the same thing that never worked before and expecting different results.) Then she found people with love and wisdom—Alcoholics Anonymous—who have been helping people to recover from "mental illness" and drugs for more than fifty years and who taught her how to grow up and be a psychological adult. Smith is now executive director of Welcome World, Inc., a tax-deductible nonprofit group for public awareness that maintains that in life, as in any business or endeavor, if the person does not have the needed mental tools, what works is to teach that person the needed mental tools.

Dee dee Bloom, a resident of Juneau, Alaska, finds her spiritual home with Pele on the Big Island of Hawaii. Surviving ritual violence and later psychotherapy and psychiatric assault led her to explore the relationship between dominant religious, military, medical, and economic theories and practices. She now works and teaches in healing arts and sciences considered "questionable" by those in power. At 45 she began her formal study of homeopathic healing, adding yet another beautiful gift to her medicine bag.

Dorothy Washburn Dundas is a graduate of Boston University. She has been a freelance writer for more than fifteen years, with a special interest in writing op-ed pieces that expose the human rights violations within the mental health system. She lives with her four children in Newton, Massachusetts.

Elaine Erickson received a Master of Music degree in music composition from Drake University in 1967. She has since studied music at Peabody Conservatory in Baltimore, Maryland. While there she wrote four operas, three of which were performed at Peabody. She has had four books of poems, including *Solo Drive* and *Portraits and Selected Poems*, published by Chestnut Hills Press in Baltimore, and her poems have been published in numerous journals. Now she teaches music composition at Central College in Pella, Iowa, and lives in Des Moines with her cat, Flora.

Janet Foner is a former full-time painter and printmaker with a master's degree in community psychology. Married and the mother of two boys aged 17 and 22, she is co-coordinator of Support Coalition International, an international coalition of groups for human rights in psychiatry. Foner is also the International Liberation Reference Person for Mental Health System Survivors in Reevaluation Counseling and has led many workshops in the U.S. and Canada. She reports, "I have never been happier in my life than while working with psychiatric survivors for our liberation. We are an unstoppable, wonderful, warm and dynamic bunch of people."

Janet Gotkin, survivor of both psychiatry and incest, is coauthor (with her husband, Paul) of *Too Much Anger, Too Many Tears: A Personal Triumph Over Psychiatry.*

Janice L. Norman is a consumer information specialist, researcher, and writer. She is a legal consultant on disability issues, especially on the abuse called psychiatry. She thanks her family, friends, and the New England Baha'i Community for questioning and fighting the abuse and insanity of psychiatry.

Jeanine Grobe is a pianist/teacher, writer, artist, and psychiatric survivor. She reports, "I am passionate about life and pursue everything I'm drawn to. It's harder for psychiatry to hit a moving target."

Jodi Lundgren writes, dances, teaches and wears purple on the West Coast of Canada, where the ocean sustains her spirit.

Judi Chamberlin has been an activist in the psychiatric inmates' liberation movement since 1971. She is a founding member of the Ruby Rogers Advocacy and Drop-In Center in Cambridge, Massachusetts, and the National Association of Psychiatric Survivors. She will continue her activism until no one can be forced into the psychiatric system against her will, and until voluntary, self-help alternatives are available for all who want them.

Kris Yates is a 43-year-old lesbian raised in Tennessee by a single mother who went to the ninth grade. Getting her M.A. in 1994 was an important achievement for Yates. However, she reports, "my greatest accomplishment was surviving electroshock in

India in my twenties. Time in nature, using my body, loving myself and others well, and activism have all helped me heal."

Lorelee Stewart is executive director of The Independent Living Center of the North Shore in Lynn, Massachusetts. She served for two years as the external vice president of the National Council on Independent Living and is a member of the National Association of Psychiatric Survivors. Stewart has a dissociative disorder and uses Personal Assistance Services to live and work in the community. Lorelee speaks on this issue across the country. She has also written and published several articles.

Margaret Robison is author of *The Naked Bear* (Lynx House Press/Panache, 1977) and *Red Creek* (Amherst Writers and Artists Press, 1992). Before having a stroke that paralyzed her left side, she served as a Poet-In-Residence in Massachusetts schools, and taught women in prison. Now she leads a writing workshop for women with disabilities. Her work has been published in journals such as *Kaleidoscope, Disability Rag, Sinister Wisdom,* and *Yankee Magazine.*

Myra Lilliana Splitrock defines herself as "a white lesbian Artist writer growing toward loving all. I left Europe gradually. In the past eight years I've managed OASIS, a space for women in Teponltan. I'm now in Guadalajara, Mexico, and its liveliness has helped me heal and grow. I'm mostly in the closet about being an ex mental patient. My plants and doggy keep me in the present."

Myrna Renner is a 47-year-old mental hospital survivor— physical abuse and incest survivor—still within the mental health system. She loves writing poetry and short stories. She reports, "My greatest passion is my freedom to be in the outside world and walk in the sun, instead of darkness."

Rae Unzicker is a writer, speaker, and consultant who has told her personal story in more than thirty states, as well as on all the major television talk shows, and frequently consults with the Center for Mental Health Services. She has been involved in the ex-patients' movement for more than fifteen years and was one of the founding members of the National Association of Psychiatric Survivors. She also serves on the board of directors of the National Association for Rights Protection and Advocacy.

Index

246

We gratefully acknowledge the following for permission to reprint previously published work:

BATYA WEINBAUM: "The 13th State" appeared in *Phoenix Rising*, vol. 2, no. 3, 1981. Reprinted by permission of the author and Phoenix Rising.

BATYA WEINBAUM: "A Woman on Society's Terms" appeared in *Big Mama Rag*, May 1982. Reprinted by permission of the author.

BLUEBIRD: "For Children Who Keep Banging" appeared in *Dare To Vision*, Holyoke, MA: Human Resources Association of the Northeast, 1994. Reprinted by permission of the author.

BETTY BLASKA: "What it is Like to be Treated Like a CMI" appeared in *Schizophrenia Bulletin*, vol. 17, no. 1, 1991. Reprinted by permission of the author.

CATHARINE ODETTE: "Suicide: A Verb" appeared in *Dykes, Disability and Stuff*, vol. 3, no. 1. Reprinted by permission of the author.

CLOVER: "Psychiatry Nitty Gritty" appeared in *Communiqué*, the Foothills Art Center Newsletter. Reprinted by permission of the author.

DEE DEE BLOOM: "Money Changes Everything" appeared in *Sinister Wisdom 36*, Winter 1988-1989. Reprinted by permission of the author.

ELAINE ERICKSON: "Madwoman" and "Insomniac" appeared in *Solo Drive*, Baltimore, MD: Chestnut Hills Press, 1992; and *Portraits and Selected Poems*, Baltimore, MD: Chestnut Hills Press, 1994. Reprinted by permission of the author.

JANICE L. NORMAN: "A Refugee in My Own Country" appeared in *Voices*, Westhampton, MA: Pine Island Press, 1990. Reprinted by permission of the author.

JUDI CHAMBERLIN: "Struggling to be Born" appeared in *Women Look at Psychiatry*, Dorothy E. Smith and Sara J. David, eds., Vancouver, BC: Press Gang Publishers, 1975. Reprinted by permission of the author.

MARGARET ROBISON: "Signs" appeared in *SLANT*, Summer 1991. Reprinted by permission of the author.

MARGARET ROBISON: "Because of These Things" appeared in *Sinister Wisdom 36*, winter 1988-1989. Reprinted by permission of the author.

RAE UNZICKER: "The 'E' Word" appeared in *The Rights Tenet*, Autumn 1993. Reprinted by permission of the author.

Other Books from Third Side Press

NOVELS

Entwined   by Beatrice Stone.   Lottie Mower was put into the Lima State Hospital when she was 20 years old and remained there for 47 years years. When young Charly Simpson meets her, she is 77 and living in a nursing home where she rarely speaks. Charly, unable to learn much about Lottie from the medical records, begins dreaming Lottie's young life and wondering whether she's going crazy too. A novel of the triumph of the human spirit.

.